Contei

Introduction

Ever felt like your body is staging a rebellion, turning against you in ways you never expected? Welcome to the club – the menopause club, and this book is your friendly guide to navigate its winding road. It will equip you with the knowledge to understand what's happening in your body, practical strategies to manage symptoms, and the motivation to embrace this transition positively. By the end of this book, you will feel informed, empowered, and ready to take charge!

As I begin, it's important to point out that the time of menopause, for many women, marks a wonderful new part of life - once you get over the peri menopause and the early stages and there are lots of ways that you can do this!

One of the things I hear a lot about, and not just about women, is that we 'live much longer these days' and as a result we experience more 'problems with age' with the implication being that we are not designed to live as long as we do. When this is tied to menopause, as it often is, this becomes "women aren't supposed to live too much longer after childbirth" and that is why "menopause is now such a big issue".

These ideas are based on the belief that 'we live longer today', and that 'nature had designed the role of women to reproduce' and nothing else.

As I take an unexpected turn here, bear with me, because I am about to talk about whales. It is not a reference to weight gain - I cover that later, and don't worry about it! It's normal, natural and manageable.

Female Orcas are one of the few, if not only, species other than humans that experience menopause. In Orcas, menopause occurs when females reach their late 30s or early 40s, after which they can no longer reproduce. This is believed to offer an evolutionary advantage.

Orcas live in tight-knit family groups, which you will know as a pod, and they are typically led by the oldest female orca, often a grandmother or great-grandmother. This matriarchal structure is common amongst Orcas and has been observed in lots of studies.

The matriarch plays a crucial role in the survival of the pod, as she has extensive knowledge of hunting techniques, food sources, and migration routes. This information is passed down through the generations, and is crucial to survival, ensuring the continued success of the pod.

The reasons behind menopause in orcas are not completely understood, but one widely accepted theory is the "grandmother hypothesis."

This hypothesis suggests that older female Orcas, no longer able to reproduce, shift their focus to helping their children and grandchildren survive. These post-reproductive females contribute valuable knowledge and resources to their family groups, increasing the survival rates of their family and wider orca community.

As I point to an example from nature of the vital importance of post-reproductive females to her community's survival I also want to remind you of our history, and one that I have written about when it comes to herbal medicine.

Long before the patriarchal society, women gathered herbs and plants to provide for the family, providing not only medicine, but also the protein that the family needed to survive. They often did this with other women, and in the process learned to share their knowledge with each other - in other words they learned to communicate. This meant that they shared the food they were using, where they found it, and what plants to use for what illness. Men were not doing this. They couldn't. They were the hunter for another type of protein and communicating during hunting would have not helped catch an animal. But, vitally, meat protein would sometimes have been scarce, and so sharing any information of where it could be found would not always have been in their interests. This meant that it was women who began to create language and society, and eventually, as they learned to grow their plants, they set the seeds - literally - of farming and homesteading. It is from here that animal husbandry could begin, ending with the society structures that we know today. But during this time and for generations to follow, women shared their knowledge, particularly of medicines and food and without it, we would not have survived.

And they did this long after ending their reproductive years. We now know that humans lived into their 70's and 80's much the same as we do today (although today, for the first time in history we are not living as long as we have done in the past, due more to lifestyle and how are foods are made and the air that we breath - but that is another story).

The reason this is so confusing is the use of the term 'life expectancy' rather than 'lifetime'. Life expectancy is an average of the population. In years gone by many, many more people (both mothers and children) died at childbirth or from disease, war, or number of other reasons that don't effect us in the same way today. This meant that many died much younger than we do now for these reasons alone - not because of some 'problem' with the capabilities of our bodies. We now have evidence that, for those that avoided illness, they lived into their 70's and 80's and this was the case thousands of years ago. To make this easier to understand, if the total population was 10, and 5 died in child-birth (age o) and 5 died at 100, the 'life expectancy' would be 50 years, although a 'lifetime' was a 100 years.

I say all of this to point out that menopause is not only natural, but that it is a vital part of life - and we can do so much with our lives as we reach the mid-point. And that we are natu-rally capable of doing so. If you feel a sense of loss or grief, or feel old or useless, as you reach this phase of your life, try not to. Try to remember our grandmothers and our grandmothers before them - they are the ones who built the societies, and the knowledge, that we still depend upon today.

But first, we need to get through it! And this is what this book is about - it's a simple tool to use that explains what is going on, why it is happening and what you can do about it.

I am 56 years old, and at the time I as entering peri menopause, I still had little-to-no knowledge about hormones and a lack of awareness of what was happening, and what I could, or should, do about it. This was probably around 10 years ago and, even at that time, therapies like HRT and estrogen replacement were believed to be 'dangerous'.

They are not, and especially not today. There are also lots of other strategies that you can use to help support your hormones, and your mental and body health at this time if you can't, or don't want to, use HRT - and they will go on to help you in later life too.

90% of women will experience at least some symptoms of menopause, and for the 10% who don't, this is because they are still producing some testosterone in their adrenal glands and some estrogen in their fat. We talk about this later. Even if you don't think you have had any symptoms - read on, because you might be surprised to discover that indeed you have.

I am not a Doctor, but even if I was, it's possible I would

know less than I do now. I have read books, poured over research, been on courses and read hundreds of reports - because I had to. There was no other way to find answers. I spoke to a Doctor just last week, a great guy and a very good doctor, and as we talked about menopause and the support options, I was surprised how closely he listened, before realising that I knew more than he did - and he was happy to let me know this. Even today, we still need to be our own experts.

I went to see my local GP at various times during those early years, and not once, did he (and sometimes she) suggest my problems might be menopausal. I now know that at least some of them were. I went back to another doctor much later because I was a losing my hair and by this time I knew it had to be hormone related. He prescribed Vitamin D (and didn't bother to check my calcium intake) - and appeared either reluctant to tackle the issue of hormones or unaware that this might be the cause of my symptoms.

Hormones effect different women in different ways and there is no truer an example of this than the menopause. Some women appear to sail through it with few symptoms while others experience a range of issues that can have a severe impact on day-to-day living. Estimates of the number of symptoms range from 26 to 96 and this should give you an idea of the broad ranging impact of our hormones on our health.

Just as this is true of the symptoms, the solutions and the support that can be provided will vary from woman-to-woman. We will all react to reducing hormones in different ways and with it, how we individually respond to the changing levels and imbalances.

A great example of this is estrogen replacement therapy or HRT. Some women might use HRT for many years, some might choose to use it over the first years of the menopause whilst others either might choose, or can't, use it at all.

The reasons are varied - some worry about using it too long.

This can be because they feel that lowering estrogen levels are a natural part of life's cycle and that the sooner their body gets used to it the better. Some might be concerned about longer term health impacts such as cancer (HRT is safe in the vast majority of cases), and there are women who can't use HRT for a number of health reasons. There are also women who feel that their symptoms are having such a dramatic effect on their life that the sooner they can access HRT the better.

At the end of the day, it's a personal choice. But I can't help wondering about the impact that the an infamous research paper had all those years ago, yet that still gets quoted again today, as the underlying reason for women choosing not to use HRT. I will cover HRT in its own dedicated chapter to help shine more light on what it is and why it can help but also cover other remedies and natural support that can be used.

For women, the most significant cause of many of the effects of the hormonal changes, especially before and during menopause is lowering estrogen and progesterone levels (and to a lesser degree, testosterone) and imbalance this causes across a variety of other hormones as well as the parts of our body systems that they communicate with. It impacts on our heart health, our mental health, all the way to our bones, skin, hair and nails and then on to the longer term impacts of osteoporosis and alzhiemer's. All of these are mainly caused by the action that estrogen and progesterone has, be it on their own or because of how it works within our body and our other hormones.

Understanding these can mean that you can support your body in specific ways. Either through HRT, supplements, diet, exercise and of also even herbs.

There are no herbs that can replace estrogen in the body and the protein it provides, but there are many, some very similar, that can help alleviate some of the problems that you might experience.

It is for this reason that exploring what is happening in your body, and why, can help identify what you can do to support it.

Whatever you decide, there is no doubt that dealing with your hormone levels and understanding them can not only help you navigate the menopause journey, but it can also significantly improve your quality of life as you age.

It really is important to remember that we are all different and what works for one person, may not work as well for another. We all have a different health make-up and so try to find out, and explore, what works for you, and what the underlying cause of any problem might be. I will outline some tests later in the book that you might want to consider.

For now, I will try and introduce you to what this book is about.

Hormones are perhaps one of our most vital life systems. They are extremely clever and they travel around our body using the endocrine superhighway, communicating with almost every part of our body, from our systems to our nerves to our organs. Their job is to keep our body in balance so that we operate efficiently and healthily. I believe hormone imbalance is one of the fundamental causes of many health problems including the problems that come with hormone imbalance during menopause. But while I know that more information is needed for women, I also know that it is also needed for men too. Look around and whenever men's health comes up it is usually around fitness and exercise, but where do men's hormones fit it? Any they must. But that subject is for another book, and here, in this book, I will only focus on women's hormones.

This is because, for women, the impact of hormones on health touches almost every aspect of life, particularly at the time of peri-menopause and menopause when we either stop producing hormones, or produce less of them. This can begin from as early as our early thirties, and all the way into our fifties, sixties and possibly even seventies.

For all women this reduction in hormone levels will impact their health - even if you don't think that it has, or that it will, it is inescapable.

The beginning of the book talks about hormones and how our body works. This means that, not only can we work out how we might be able to support our body, but knowing the why allows us to reduce our anxiety by making us feel more in control. This, in itself, can help. Anxiety is a real condition and, it too, effects our body.

One of the biggest mis-understanding centres around mood swings, anger, low energy and a feeling of 'depression'. It is not a depression in the normal sense, and it is not one that anti-depressants can 'fix'. There is a reason that you feel like you do and there are many ways that you can manage the worst of it naturally.

Another very common symptom of our hormones changes is, of course, night sweats and hot flashes or flushes, and then painful joints and hair loss. But did you know that science now proves that heart problems and osteoporosis can be 'helped' by managing hormonal balance early? Or that alzheimers in now also thought to be worse for women because of hormonal change? These are long-term conditions that are directly effected by the loss of hormones during peri-menopause and menopause that will go on to have major influences on your life as you age, changing your quality of life. If there is something that you can do that will help - even if it 'might' help, would you do it? And one that has no known risks if done in consultation with a medical professional?

Even the shorter term effects on life quality and mental health are not to be understated. They can be significant for many women. So significant in fact, that suicide amongst women is higher between the ages of 50-60 than at any other time, and higher than men.

Here are just some of the comments women have said to me.

"I remember one day leaving the house and a woman at the end of my path did something that annoyed me. I was out of control in my response, and in a way that I had never been before. It shocked me. I went to the doctor and he gave me anti-depressants".

"I cried a lot. I would get frustrated and then burst into tears. I was diagnosed as being depressed. I thought I was depressed!"

"I hated the night sweats. I hated staying with people because at home I could get up and change the sheets which I did almost every night - sometimes twice a night."

"I used to get really embarrassed at work when I would suddenly became flushed, sweaty and very hot. My solution was to always wear shirts with short sleeves."

"I couldn't understand why I put so much weight on, and no matter what I did or what I ate, it just got worse. I felt a failure."

"I was losing my hair and I was only 50, it became an obsession for me, and I didn't even want to shower or wash my hair because I couldn't bear to look at the plug hole afterwards- it was always full of my hair. I spoke to my Doctor and he gave me Vitamin D. I had no idea why."

"I woke up with my heart racing and I was so anxious - I don't know why"

The purpose of this book is to empower you with the knowledge and tools to achieve hormonal balance and optimal health – naturally if at all possible but not exclusively.

By understanding the role of hormones and how they impact our bodies, we can make informed choices about our diet, lifestyle, and health practices which can improve our energy levels, mood, sleep, and overall quality of life.

The first part of the book is all about the effects of our hormonal changes and what is happening to our body.

In the second part of the book we will also look at many of

the most common symptoms and problems that you might experience and include a range of things you can do to improve them.

Many can be helped with herbs, diet and lifestyle but also HRT, and in the final part of the book I talk about the strategies you can use to minimise the impact menopause can have on your life so that you can enjoy some of the best years of your life. You really don't need to suffer. But more than this, you can protect your longer term health too.

In terms of HRT - this is all about estrogen, progesterone replacement, and often testosterone. Almost every condition can be helped by these hormones - the ones we loose during peri-menopause and menopause.

Estrogen, progesterone and testosterone are the hormones which regulate our menstrual cycle and support the body and the unborn child during pregnancy. But they also do a lot of other things that support women's health. Estrogen , for example, as well as regulating the menstrual cycle and reproductive health, promotes bone and skin health and affects mood and cognitive function (memory loss, brain 'fog' and so on).

These three hormones are not the only hormones effected but they are the main protagonists.

What you will notice throughout the book is the role that estrogen, in particular, plays in so many of our body systems either directly or indirectly because of how it works with other hormones. By knowing which elements are being reduced or restricted by the lowering estrogen levels we can then have an idea of what might help with some of the symptoms.

Just remember that all women will eventually undergo menopause and there is a large variation in not only age, but each woman's experience of its how it impacts their health as well as mental health and well-being. I hope that the following pages not only describe the most common effects, but provide the information you need to help you navigate the experience so that it is not something that you 'need to get through' but that arms you with the tools so that you can continue to enjoy the best of times. And they really can be the best of times!

One last point of note. In this book I use the spelling estrogen. It is the most common spelling in the US and is easier to write! In Canada, the UK and Australia the correct spelling is oestrogen - I hope you forgive me.

Part I: Understanding Menopause and Hormones

ONE

The Three-Stage Symphony of Menopause

I f you don't quite know what perimenopause or menopause is, then don't worry you are not alone. And if you aren't fully aware of all of the symptoms and effects it can have, you are likely to be one of most women.

Remarkably few or us realise the broad ranging impact the drop in hormones can have on our body and our mind. And, for most doctors and physicians, who were not taught about it in medical school, they too, are catching up.

It's worth having at least a general knowledge of what's going on and in the following chapter we will set the stage of how our menstrual cycle works and what the menopause actually is.

But first what does the menopause mean?

Simply put, it is the pausing of the menstrual cycle or in other words, when women stop producing eggs. Females of reproductive age have cycles of hormonal activity that repeat at about one-month intervals or 28 days. Until the peri menopause.

An ovulatory and an anovulatory cycle

The four main hormones that regulate the activity of cells or organs in the menstrual cycle include Estrogen, Progesterone, Follicle-stimulating hormone (FSH), and Luteinizing hormone (LH). As you research your hormone journey you will hear about all of these hormones.

The central point at which everything centres is ovulation - which happens in the middle of the 28 day cycle. During the first 14 days you make more estrogen (estradiol) than progesterone, and, after ovulation, you make more progesterone than estrogen. An ovulatory cycle is when you make both progesterone and estrogen and ovulation has occurred.

An anovulatory cycle means no ovulation occurs and no progesterone was made - this is because progesterone is only made a result of ovulation. It means that after menopause you don't make progesterone. It is also the anovulatory cycle that is most common during peri menopause.

Follicular phase: This phase begins on the first day of your period and during this phase estrogen is released by the ovaries causing the the lining of the uterus to thicken as it builds up with blood and nutrients in anticipation of receiving a fertilized egg.

The follicle-stimulating hormone (FSH) and luteinizing hormone (LH) are released from the brain and travel in the blood to the ovaries where they stimulate the growth of eggs in the ovaries (which are 'cased' in a follicle). They also trigger the production of more estrogen to limit, or balance, the number of follicles. Over time, one follicle in one ovary becomes dominant and continues to produce estrogen, which stimulates the luteinizing hormone surge. This phase typically last 13 to 14 days, less nearer menopause.

Ovulatory phase (ovulation): The ovulatory phase normally begins around 14 days after the start of the follicular phase and as the levels of luteinizing hormone (LH) surge, ending with the release of the egg from the ovary (around 10-12 hours after the luteinizing surge) into the fallopian tube. The egg then travels down the fallopian tube towards the uterus (which has been getting prepared for receiving it during the follicular and luteal phase). The egg can be fertilised for up to 12 hours following release.

Luteal phase: The luteal phase begins immediately following ovulation. The, now empty, dominant follicle develops into something called the corpus luteum, which releases the hormones estrogen and progesterone and much higher levels of progesterone (compared to estrogen) is released at this time . The progesterone prepares the uterus for a fertilized egg and helps maintain the thickened uterine lining. The increase in estrogen and progesterone also dilates the milk ducts in the breasts.

If the egg is fertilized, it will travel through the fallopian tube to the uterus and implant. It is in the uterus that the baby will grow, and during the cycle it is preparing to for this task.

If the egg is not fertilized, the corpus luteum breaks down, leading to a drop in progesterone. This drop triggers the shedding of the uterine lining, which is expelled from the body as menstrual flow, marking the start of a new cycle.

Simply put, during menopause, the ovaries stop releasing eggs and significantly reduce their production of estrogen and progesterone and, in general, the timings tend to go in phases. Because progesterone is only produced during the luteal phase i.e. after ovulation, when ovulation stops as menopause officially begins, so does progesterone production.

Just because we stop producing progesterone and produce much less estrogen doesn't mean we don't retain some of their benefits. Every time we have a menstrual cycle during our life, we are adding to our 'bank' and this is what can still support our health long after we have stopped making it.

Unveiling Perimenopause

The first signs will come in early peri menopause when you start to experience irregular periods.

This phase usually begins anywhere after the age of 40 and before your monthly cycles top altogether - peri means before. It is the transitional stage leading up to menopause, marked by hormonal fluctuations and changes in menstrual patterns when you may notice changes in how heavy your periods are, and their frequency.

An average period can last between three and eight days, with the average being five and you may notice that your periods become shorter or longer during perimenopause.

Late perimenopause is most common in your late 40s or early 50s. Your periods will become further apart, and, on average, it will come every 35 days or less in your ten final cycles. The longer you go between periods, the closer you are to menopause and, eventually you will notice your periods occurring around once every 3 months before you will go 12 months without a period.

When you have gone a year without a cycle that you are in the stage of menopause. This phase can last for a decade. If you experience bleeding after this stage you may be postmenopausal bleeding and this too needs to be checked by a doctor.

Estrogen, progesterone (and, to a lesser degree, testosterone) fluctuate wildly during peri-menopause, and it is the imbalance and falls in levels of these hormones that effect our mood, anxiety, sleep, bones, mental health, weight and so on - more-or-less all of the experiences you will have to some degree or another before, during and after menopause.

Do not under-estimate the peri-menopause. It is not a gentle introduction to the menopause, not by a long chalk. Your hormones are fluctuating wildly, your PMS (irritability, mood swings etc) often gets worse and rather lasting for a day or two it continues for much longer. But there is much more to it than this.

Your periods might be either heavier or lighter, they can be closer together or further apart and for many women they can be a real problem. Not only unpredictable, but some women experience severe bleeding, which can not only be embarrassing, but prevent you from going out, and in more occasions than you might think, it can make you dread going to work, often avoiding it, and in some cases, giving it up all together.

This is also the time when you might make big decisions, then wonder about them years later. It is when you may split up from your partner, get divorced (in the UK around 60% of divorces are instigated by women and this tends to be most common between the age of 45-49), or radically change your life. Sometimes it can be for the better. Meanwhile, some women discover other women for the first time and fall in love, others discover the career they have always wanted. But for many women this is the time where anxiety levels dramatically rise, night sweats bring sleepless nights, depression kicks in and it is also the time that some women commit suicide.

For black women, the peri-menopause can start much earlier. This is not fully understood and much more research is needed because the impact of peri-menopause and menopause is not the same across all women, regions and ethnicity. In Japan for example, while the age of menopause is broadly similar (50 to 52 years old) it is widely reported that women experience milder menopausal symptoms compared to their Western counterparts. It has been theorised that the reason for this is a soy-based diet. Soy is a source of body-identical hormones, which I go on to talk about later.

To understand what all this means in terms of the peri menopause and the menopause we need to go back to your teenage years.

Estrogen starts to increase as you reach puberty and becomes high during your teens. Progesterone starts to slowly rise as your periods begin and, as your cycle becomes established, progesterone also reaches high levels. But it is the phase when you have higher levels of estrogen compared to the lower levels of progesterone that can cause heavier periods during puberty.

When you begin the peri-menopause progesterone levels slowly drop, also giving you high estrogen levels compared to progesterone. Once again, it is this which can cause heavy bleeding during your period.

Eventually your estrogen levels 'catch up' giving you low levels of both hormones (and lower levels of testosterone) which brings you back to a similar level to where you started pre puberty.

As we have touched on, the reason this impacts our health is that this reduction in egg production means that less hormones are produced - particularly estrogen, progesterone and testosterone. As well as regulating our menstrual cycle and supporting the body during pregnancy, these hormones have a vital role to play in our overall health and well-being.

As estrogen and progesterone levels fall, women may experience symptoms such as hot flashes, night sweats, mood swings, vaginal dryness, and sleep disturbances. These hormonal changes can also contribute to an increased risk of osteoporosis and cardiovascular disease. We will cover all of these, and others, over the course of this book.

Menopause in Full Swing

Menopause itself is a point in time marking 12 months since your last menstrual period but the symptoms and hormonal fluctuations surrounding menopause can last for several years - and occasionally as long as 15-20 years. If this has just happened, its useful to know that you can still get pregnant before the menopause starts, even towards the end of perimenopause, so if there is any chance of this, take a pregnancy test!

The symptoms and effects are wide-raging and can include weight gain, sleeplessness, mood swings, feelings similar to depression, heart palpations, heart attack, along with hair loss (and growth!), lumpy sore breasts, urine problems and vaginal dryness along with aggy skin. Last, but not least, it can cause painful bones and joints along with a lack of - or non-existent - libido.

Postmenopause refers to the years after menopause, where hormonal levels stabilize and symptoms may continue or subside.

The long-term effects of menopause on your health, include bone density loss and increased risk of heart disease

If supported at that time (and 7-10 years after onset) the impact on health and well-being can be smoothed and helped by knowing what your body needs for support.

The causes are simple - hormone changes. And the effect of these hormone changes can be supported and helped along for many of not most of the conditions. Better still, the solutions are easy. There really is no need today, to suffer and it is this, and these symptoms that we cover in the following chapters.

The Hysterectomy and Oophorectomy

Before we go on to the effects of hormone loss, it is important to point out that some women may need to have their uterus (hysterectomy) or ovaries (oophorectomy) removed at a young age, and this can be for many reasons.

As we know, the ovaries are responsible for producing estrogen and progesterone. While the removal of the ovaries has the effect of inducing menopause, the removal of the uterus will mean that hormones are still being produced but that it won't be possible to have a baby. The choice between removing the uterus, the ovaries, or both depends on the specific condition and overall health. For example, if a woman has uterine cancer but her ovaries are healthy, she may only need a hysterectomy. If she has ovarian cancer, an oophorectomy might be necessary. If both organs are affected, or if there's a high risk of cancer due to genetic factors, both might be removed.

The surgical removal of the uterus (hysterectomy), does not typically cause menopause symptoms immediately after the procedure, as long as the ovaries are left in place. This is because the ovaries are the organs responsible for producing most of the hormones (estrogen and progesterone) that regulate the menstrual cycle and impact menopause symptoms.

There are a few ways that a hysterectomy can eventually lead to menopause or menopause-like symptoms:

Indirect Impact: Some women may experience a decrease in ovarian function after a hysterectomy, even if the ovaries are not removed. This could potentially lead to earlier onset of menopause, but this is still a subject of ongoing research.

Ovarian Failure: If a woman has a hysterectomy and one or both of her ovaries are removed (an oophorectomy), she will experience what's often called "surgical menopause." The sudden drop in estrogen and progesterone levels caused by the removal of the ovaries can lead to immediate and severe menopause symptoms.

No More Periods: After a hysterectomy, a woman will no longer have menstrual periods. While this is not the same as menopause (which involves changes in hormone levels), it can be seen as a symptom similar to post-menopause when periods naturally stop.

Prophylactic Oophorectomy: In some cases, a woman may choose to have her ovaries removed at the time of hysterectomy to prevent ovarian cancer, especially if she has a high risk due to genetic factors. This will also lead to surgical menopause.

Early menopause, which effects 1 in 100 women, typically refers to menopause occurring before the age of 45 and when it's been a year since the last period. Premature Ovarian Insufficiency (POI), effects closer to 1 in 1000 women, and is when menopause occurs before the age of 40 - and it can be as early as 30.

The Prima Ballerina: Estrogen

Estrogen regulates the menstrual cycle, and is best known for supporting reproductive health. Less well known is its role in maintaining bone density, its impact on mood, skin and vaginal health, as well as cardiovascular health. It has lots of other benefits that are highlighted throughout the following pages.

Symptoms of an estrogen deficiency range from hot flashes, vaginal dryness, and mood swings - so take note if you experience any of these and they can occur after the onset of menopause as well as during peri menopause. Sometimes vaginal dryness can only become a problem well into your sixties (topical estrogen can help and has almost no known side effects - this topic has its own chapter).

Estradiol, estrone, and estriol are the three main types of estrogen hormones, and they differ in their potency, functions, and where they are produced.

Estradiol (E2) is the most potent and prevalent estrogen hormone, mainly produced in the ovaries. It has a significant role in regulating the menstrual cycle, developing female secondary sexual characteristics, maintaining bone health, and influencing mood and cognitive function. This is the type of estrogen most commonly referred to when it comes to menopause 'estrogen' and is the the type that will usually be referred to during the following pages and chapters.

Estrone (E1) is weaker than estradiol, and it, too, is produced in the ovaries, but it can also be converted from estradiol in the liver and from androstenedione (a precursor to estrogen and testosterone) in fat tissue.

Estrone is the main form of estrogen in postmenopausal women, but only because the production of estradiol declines after menopause, not because estrone levels have increased. Estrone still contributes to bone health and other estrogen-related functions but at a reduced level compared to estradiol.

Estriol (E3) is the weakest of the three main estrogens. It is produced in significant amounts during pregnancy, mainly by the placenta. Estriol levels rise throughout pregnancy, reaching their highest levels just before birth, and it is thought to help prepare the body for childbirth. In non-pregnant individuals, estriol is present at much lower levels and has a minimal impact on estrogen-related functions compared to estradiol and estrone.

There are many symptoms caused be falling estrogen levels and they are different for all women. We cover most of the common ones in the following chapters, including dry mouth, heart palpitations, hair loss, itchy skin, dry eyes, vaginal dryness, dizziness, brain fog, sore joints, low energy, anxiety, short temper, and feelings of depression. Women are also more prone to osteoporosis, arthritis, calcification (where the calcium builds on the outside of the bone), and heart-related issues.

Short-term symptoms include hot flashes, night sweats, sleep disturbances, and mood swings. These are mainly caused by a lack of estrogen because of its thermoregulatory effect on the body.

As estrogen reduces, it can cause sudden changes in body temperature, and it is this that results in the hot flashes and night sweats. It also regulates the levels and actions of neurotransmitters in the brain which can influence various brain functions, such as mood, sleep, cognition, and behaviour. (Nerve health is also looked after by testosterone - it protects the myelin sheath and supports the neurotransmitters).

A decline in estrogen levels has been linked to increased bone resorption and decreased bone formation, which can lead to a higher risk of osteoporosis which we cover in the chapter on bone health.

It also has protective effects on the cardiovascular system. It helps protect your heart and blood vessels by the widening or relaxing of blood vessels, which can lower blood pressure and improve blood flow. It prevents blood platelets from clumping together and forming blood clots, which can reduce the risk of heart attacks and strokes. These protective effects also help to maintain a healthy circulatory system.

Cognitive decline is another long-term concern again related to its neuroprotective effects. Although a decline in estrogen may be associated with an increased risk of Alzheimer's, more research is needed to fully understand the relationship between menopause, estrogen, and cognitive function.

I cover much of what you can do to support estrogen (and your other hormones and symptoms) throughout this book but as an example here, lifestyle changes and dietary choices that can help support estrogen production and balance. For example, incorporating phytoestrogen-rich foods into your diet, such as soy, flaxseeds, and legumes and engaging in regular physical activity can help to support estrogen production and overall well-being.

The Supporting Cast: Progesterone

As we know progesterone is another crucial hormone involved in the menstrual cycle and pregnancy. It works in tandem with estrogen to regulate the menstrual cycle and prepare the body for potential pregnancy. It's job it to counteract the uterine thickening of estrogen and is one of the reason's why it helps guard against heavy periods.

Progesterone builds bones, boosts energy, helps sleep, soothes mood, boosts hair and skin, lightens periods, and thins the womb lining (helping to prevent uterine cancer), is great for urinary

health and you make a lot of it - in fact, we make more progesterone than we do estrogen.

In the second half of the cycle, the luteal phase (after ovulation), progesterone levels rise. This means that if you are not
ovulating, you can't make progesterone because it is only
produced after ovulation.

Progesterone levels decline during peri menopause because
the ovaries are producing less of this hormone (whereas, at this
time estrogen levels remain 'high' in comparison). Low progesterone levels can contribute to insomnia, anxiety, and mood
swings.

In peri menopause, when progesterone and estrogen are out
of balance and when you have more estrogen relative to progesterone, it can lead to symptoms including hot flashes, mood
swings, decreased libido, and heart palpitations.

If you are taking any kind of hormone replacement - either
using HRT or natural remedies and you have a uterus then you
need to take progesterone with estrogen. This is because
estrogen makes the uterine lining grow. Adding progesterone
stops this growth protecting against problems including uterine
cancer.

Cast member: Testosterone

Androgens are a group of hormones that play a crucial role in
developing and maintaining male characteristics. They are often
referred to as "male hormones," although they are also present in
women in different amounts.

Testosterone is the most well-known androgen, but there are
others, like dihydrotestosterone (DHT) and androstenedione. In
women, they are made by the ovaries and adrenal glands.

Androgens have a variety of functions in the body, including:

- Development of male reproductive organs and secondary sexual characteristics (e.g., facial hair, deepening of the voice) during puberty.
- Regulation of libido (sex drive)
- Stimulation of muscle growth and bone mass.
- Regulation of hair growth patterns.

Testosterone levels in women decline gradually with age and it is this decline that can result in a decrease in sex drive, muscle mass, and also bone density.

Interactive Exercise: Keep a diary

Some women may have an indication of how they will cope with menopause by thinking back to when they were pregnant and how they felt both during and after birth. We all operate differently, and some women, during pregnancy, feel like they are the fittest they have ever been, yet immediately after birth, they sink into post-natal depression. This could be the result of high estrogen during pregnancy and then the significant loss of estrogen following the birth of a child. But, don't rely on how you experienced pregnancy or puberty to predict your menopause symptoms.

As you lead up to peri menopause and menopause, and this can be from 40 onwards, you might notice that a few weeks before your period, you start to feel a lack of energy; you may also be experiencing night sweats and anxiety, you might be tearful and irritable, and so on. Yet once your period starts, you feel fine.

Additionally, PMS can often get worse during perimenopause and increases irritability, mood swings, and so on, and rather than lasting a day or two, it goes on for much longer.

It is essential to know your symptoms and causes as early as possible so you can support your body during peri menopause and the early years of menopause. If you do this, you can avoid many more severe conditions that can impact your life in the following years.

For those of you approaching the time of peri menopause, now is a great time to start a diary - it can prove invaluable in diagnosis. Keep track of your monthly cycle, including when your period starts and ends, and include any symptoms even if you don't think they are related (dizziness, migraines, energy levels, etc.). As with most things, the more you know, then the easier it is to diagnose, and the more that can be done.

Lastly, understanding what is happening and why can help us empathize with and support other women going through this transition. Menopause is a shared experience for women, and by knowing what's happening on a physiological, as well as on a physical level, means we can create a community of understanding, encouragement, and support for one another.

TWO

Stress, Cortisol and our Adrenal Angel

Menopause presents a unique challenge for the body as it navigates the shifting hormonal landscape, with the adrenal glands taking center stage in managing stress. As cortisol levels fluctuate, they can either be a friend or foe, making it crucial to understand and support the adrenal glands during this transformative phase of life.

P icture this: you're walking in the woods, and you suddenly come face to face with a bear. Your heart races, your palms get sweaty, and you're ready to either fight or flee. Who do you have to thank for that rapid response? Your adrenal glands.

These small, triangular-shaped glands that sit on top of your kidneys help your body manage stress and maintain energy levels. They secrete various hormones, such as cortisol, adrenaline, and aldosterone, which all help to regulate your blood pressure, immune system, and metabolism.

Cortisol the stress hormone

Cortisol, the "stress hormone", helps your body respond to stressful situations, like our bear encounter, by increasing blood sugar levels and suppressing non-essential functions, such as digestion and reproduction.

Adrenaline, on the other hand, is responsible for that rapid heart rate and surge of energy you feel when facing danger. Finally, aldosterone helps maintain a proper balance of salt and water in your body, which in turn helps regulate your blood pressure.

In short, your adrenal glands are like your body's built-in alarm system, helping you respond to threats and maintain balance in everyday life.

The impact of imbalances on adrenal health

Born in the adrenal cortex, cortisol's primary role is to prepare our bodies to confront challenges. This hormone governs our natural 'fight or flight' response, assisting us during times of stress, be it physical or emotional.

It's crucial to appreciate that its rhythm in our bodies is as critical as its overall volume. Normally, cortisol levels rise and fall, peaking in the early morning to ignite our vitality for the day's tasks, and ebbing by evening, allowing us to rest and rejuvenate.

When stress becomes a relentless shadow, our adrenals can become overworked, leading to a condition known as adrenal fatigue or adrenal dysfunction. This can result in an imbalance of hormones, such as cortisol, which may be too high or too low at various times throughout the day.

It causes sleep disturbances, fatigue and a range of other symptoms, including mood swings, difficulty concentrating, and even weight gain. In other words, adrenal dysfunction can leave you feeling utterly drained and out of sorts.

The adrenal glands, just like the all the glands in our endocrine system, communicate with through a series of feedback loops.

When we're stressed, our adrenal glands release cortisol to help us cope. This increase in cortisol can signal our bodies to release more glucose (sugar) into our bloodstream, giving us the energy we need to handle the situation. At the same time, cortisol can communicate with our immune system, telling it to slow down and take it easy so that our bodies can focus on dealing with the stressor at hand.

As we know, during menopause, our bodies go through significant hormonal changes, particularly a decline in estrogen and progesterone levels. Now, the adrenal glands are already busy producing hormones like cortisol, adrenaline, and aldosterone. But when menopause hits, they're also asked to take on the extra task of producing small amounts of estrogen and progesterone to help make up for the decline. It's like they're being asked to pick up the slack, and it can put a lot of extra pressure on them.

Here's a simple way to think about it: Imagine you're juggling three balls, and you're doing a great job. But then someone tosses in a fourth ball, and suddenly, it's much harder to keep them all in the air. That's what's happening to our adrenal glands during menopause. They're trying to juggle all their usual tasks while also dealing with the additional demands placed on them due to hormonal changes and they can't keep track of what they should be doing effectively.

To add to this, one of the ways our body tries to cope with the changes in estrogen levels is by increasing the production of cortisol. This means that as estrogen levels decline during perimenopause and menopause, cortisol levels increase making our stress response erratic as we become more sensitive to stressors. All of this can lead to our symptoms of fatigue, mood swings, and difficulty sleeping.

Additionally, although cortisol is essential for our body's

response to stress, and helping to maintain energy levels, blood sugar, and blood pressure, when cortisol levels are consistently high, it can also increase the risk of developing conditions like obesity, type 2 diabetes, and cardiovascular disease, particularly in women going through menopause (see weight gain)

Elevated cortisol levels can lead to weight gain, particularly around the abdomen, because it promotes the accumulation of fat cells in this area.

High cortisol levels can also make it more difficult for our body to regulate blood sugar effectively. Cortisol increases glucose production in the liver and reduces insulin sensitivity in cells, making it harder for the body to maintain healthy blood sugar levels. This can increase the risk of developing type 2 diabetes, especially for women experiencing menopause-related hormonal imbalances.

Increased cortisol levels can also contribute to cardiovascular disease by increasing blood pressure and causing inflammation in blood vessels. There are other ways in which menopause-related hormonal changes can increase the risk of heart disease, but high cortisol levels can add to this risk.

While high cortisol levels are often a concern during menopause due to increased stress, it's also possible for cortisol levels to drop too low, leading to adrenal insufficiency which can cause fatigue, weight loss, low blood pressure, and even life-threatening shock if left untreated. This tends not to be related to menopause but the combination of both can be very difficult.

Adrenal dysfunction can also have a significant impact on your mental health. Studies have shown that imbalanced cortisol levels are linked to mood disorders like depression and anxiety. In addition, high cortisol levels can disrupt your sleep patterns to such an extent that it leads to insomnia which heightens stress and mood issues.

It's worth noting that while adrenal fatigue is not a medically recognized diagnosis in many countries, many healthcare professionals acknowledge that chronic stress can lead to hormonal imbalances and decreased adrenal function.

There are a number of areas in which menopause and the changes in our hormones can affect adrenal health and some of them build upon the other. For example:

1. The hormonal fluctuations and symptoms experienced during peri-menopause and post-menopause can be stressful for many women. This added stress can place extra demand on the adrenal glands, leading to adrenal fatigue or dysfunction.
2. Many women experience sleep problems during peri-menopause and post-menopause due to hot flashes, night sweats, and general hormonal imbalance. Poor sleep can further strain the adrenal glands and disrupt cortisol production.
3. The hormonal changes during menopause, particularly the decrease in estrogen levels, can affect mood and increase the risk of depression and anxiety. This can also contribute to chronic stress, which, as we've discussed, can negatively impact adrenal health.

While menopause doesn't directly cause adrenal insufficiency, the stress and hormonal changes during this time can put additional strain on the adrenal glands and it's clear that supporting our adrenal function is important for our overall well-being.

There are a several things that we can do, and much of it is to do with managing stress and cortisol levels.

- Practice stress management: Incorporating techniques like deep breathing exercises, meditation, or yoga into your daily routine can help reduce stress and support your adrenal glands . Remember, it's not just about avoiding stress but learning how to manage it effectively.

- Prioritise sleep: Make sure you're getting enough rest each night (aim for 7-9 hours) and establishing a regular sleep schedule. Creating a bedtime routine and ensuring your sleep environment is dark, cool, and comfortable can also improve sleep quality.
- Avoid tea and coffee at least 2 hours before bedtime, and, if you must, take a cup of chamomile tea instead.
- Drink lots of water and stay hydrated. Water helps with digestion, nutrient absorption, and detoxification processes. Aim for at least eight glasses of water a day, more if you're active or live in a hot climate.
- Eat a balanced diet: Consuming a diet rich in whole foods, lean proteins, healthy fats, and plenty of fruits and vegetables can provide your body with the nutrients it needs to support adrenal function.
- Consider supplements: Some supplements, like vitamin C, B vitamins, and adaptogenic herbs (e.g., ashwagandha, rhodiola, black cohosh, soy, red clover, or ginseng), may help support adrenal health and balance hormone and function. You can have rhodiola and ginseng as a tea during the day.
- Stay active: Regular exercise is crucial for overall health and can help reduce stress, improve mood, and support adrenal function. Aim for at least 150 minutes of moderate aerobic activity each week, along with strength training exercises for all major muscle groups. And of course, take walks in nature - as well as providing exercise, it is known to be calming, acting to reduce stress
- The emotional challenges of menopause can be significant for many women, and it is essential to seek

support from friends, family, or a mental health professional if needed. Sharing your experiences and feelings with others can help reduce stress and improve your emotional well-being.

- (HRT) can help alleviate some of the symptoms of menopause by replacing declining estrogen levels. This can also help regulate cortisol levels and support adrenal health. This is covered in more detail in a later chapter.

Practices like acupuncture, tai chi, or massage therapy can help reduce menopause-related stress and promote relaxation, and anything that reduces stress is great for the adrenal gland.

Managing Stress and Building Resilience

- Stress management techniques: Exploring various strategies to manage and reduce stress during menopause.
- Time management and prioritization
- Stress-relieving exercises such as yoga or Tai Chi
- Setting realistic expectations and goals
- Building emotional resilience: Developing skills and habits that can help you bounce back from challenges and setbacks.
- Embracing flexibility and adaptability
- Nurturing a growth mindset
- Seeking support and building a strong support system

THREE

Anxiety to Assurance: Emotional Well-being in Menopause

L ife, generally brings with it lots of emotional challenges and at the time perimenopause hits many of us are in the full throes of work, often balancing family demands from teenage or you adult children to aging parents. Over the next few years our life structures will be changing regardless of menopause, but the hormone imbalances around the years from perimenopause can make things feel a whole lot worse.

Women who have not been depressed before are about 3 times more likely to develop depression during the menopause transition. Poor sleep, stress, negative life events, higher body mass index, smoking, and even a younger age at menopause start or being an African American woman can all increase this risk.

Depression, anxiety, and stress are very hard to handle and have a huge impact on mental health and well-being. You can feel panic, feel angry, joyless, and generally fed-up.

For some women this can lead to a sense of a lack of control over your emotions, and it can appear in unexpected ways. It can show up with a break down in tears at work, in the street, in the car, or in the convenience store. It can mean a lack of concentration which can be so bad that it, too, can lead to an inability to work.

You might feel low, worthless, easily annoyed, and easily triggered and have a chronic lack of concentration. If you are early perimenopausal watch out for these feelings a few days before you period starts (after ovulation) and as your estrogen levels fall. The decline in estrogen is the same reason you can feel this way during the phases during perimenopause in particular and into menopause.

For many, this dip in mood gets worse, as estrogen levels fall further, and for some women it can be so bad that it can lead to suicidal thoughts.

Many women will get diagnosed with depression or bi-polar disorder when in fact it is a lack of estrogen that is causing the mood swings and these feelings of depression.

It one of the reason's that it is so important to keep a journal of how you feel each month and keep a track of your emotions to establish the cause. You may not feel any better, but you will know what's going on and it makes it easier to find a solution.

I really don't want to underplay how important this is or the impact it can have on your life. Women I know, over the time of the peri menopause and early menopause lost all faith in themselves - they just did not recognise themselves anymore. Have you ever looked in a mirror and asked yourself "what changed?". Women who had been high flyers lost the belief that they were 'good enough', in fact they didn't feel 'good enough' for any job.

Along with collapsing confidence, women can lose the sense of value, of worth, of presence, and end up feeling insignificant. While this may or may not be due to the menopause, if you listen to some of these women talk who have used some kind of estrogen support (estrogen, progesterone and a little testosterone), as I have done, then many have re-discovered their old self.

Why Menopause Stirs Up the Emotional Pot

The reason for this is that all of these hormones have an effect on our brain. As they decline, we feel the impact. A great example of this is post natal depression. During pregnancy our hormones surge to intense levels. Once the baby is born, levels collapse (the ratio is close to 17:1). And thankfully, as we understand the role hormones play on our brain, we are now beginning to understand that this is what can cause post-natal depression. You are not a bad mum, or going mad, its simply a huge, and fast, drop in estrogen. It's also at this time that you might also experience night sweats, vaginal dryness, and a number of other 'menopause' symptoms.

There are a number of ways that falling estrogen effects our mood, and these are all linked to cortisol, the adrenal gland and the cognitive symptoms covered in this book. Another is the decline in the happy hormone Serotonin and this is where our gut and microbiome, and our diet can play a part. Adaptogenic herbs such as R. rosea, ginseng, and ashwagandha, all have some supporting research that shows they may help boost serotonin and improve mood. But daylight, too, increases the release of serotonin so get out in the daylight early in the morning, and as much as you can during the day.

Serotonin can be boosted synthetically too, and these are what are referred to when it comes to the antidepressants known as SSRIs and SNRIs. SSRIs (Selective serotonin reuptake inhibitors) work to keep serotonin circulating in the brain for long periods while SNRIs (Serotonin-norepinephrine reuptake inhibitors) work by keeping serotonin and norepinephrine circulating. Side effects can include headaches, nausea, insomnia and fatigue or libido problems.

The best way to improve your serotonin levels naturally is through diet, getting out in the sun (or supplementing with vitamin D when sunshine is limited), exercise, use adaptogens, and manage stress.

But often it's not about the volume of the decline, it is about the change happening, the imbalance your mind and body is trying to cope with, and make sense of. This means that too much can even be bad for you.

The obvious answer to this is to replace, or support, these hormones - even in younger women who are still having their periods.

Body-identical estrogen in, for example HRT gel, is reported as being safer than the contraceptive pill which contains synthetic progestin. All that happens is that as estrogen levels fluctuate more, and decline more as time progresses, your physician can alter the dosage and frequency.

It is still amazing how many women get prescribed some form of anti-depressant rather than been informed that hormone replacement is an option.

Women are getting prescribed antipsychotics and antidepressants all of which can have side effects and some that can make menopausal symptoms worse. Sometimes antidepressants can also lead to weight gain regardless of what you eat or how much exercise you are doing, and this can lower self esteem at a time when woman may already be more susceptible to low mood. For women, especially those in their 40's and 5o's who are feeling depressed, it is more than possible that this is due to an estrogen deficiency - and if you are using body identical estrogen then you are replacing something the body already produces which means it really is, in most cases, safe - and often safer than birth contraceptive pills that contain progestin.

Sometimes woman who have their ovaries removed but who still have a uterus are provided no hormonal support whatsoever. Yes, it is obvious that if you remove the hormone-producing ovaries then it will result in a massive drop in hormones which causes all of the associated effects, including depression. If this is you, find out about hormone support. Men, who have their testicles removed tend to get prescribed testosterone - the concept is well understood!

Chronic stress has also been linked to hormonal imbalances, including high levels of cortisol, disrupted thyroid function, and decreased levels of sex hormones like estrogen and testosterone.

Chronic stress can affect a variety of hormones in the body. One of the primary hormones that is impacted is cortisol, commonly known as the "stress hormone." We discussed this in an earlier chapter. Chronic stress can lead to consistently high levels of cortisol, which can have negative effects on the body, including weight gain, decreased immune function, and disrupted sleep.

Another hormone impacted by chronic stress is thyroid hormone. The thyroid gland produces hormones that regulate the body's metabolism and energy levels. Chronic stress can interfere with thyroid function, leading to imbalances in thyroid hormone levels and potentially causing symptoms such as fatigue, weight gain, and mood changes.

Falling estrogen and progesterone can also be affected by chronic stress and can lead to menstrual irregularities, fertility issues, and other health concerns.

In addition to cortisol, thyroid hormones, and our sex hormones, chronic stress can also impact insulin, the hormone responsible for regulating blood sugar levels. High levels of stress can lead to insulin resistance, which can contribute to the development of type 2 diabetes.

A study published in the Journal of Women's Health supports these effects. It found that women who reported high levels of stress also had higher levels of cortisol and lower levels of estrogen and progesterone, suggesting a potential link between chronic stress and hormonal imbalances in women. The study also found that women who participated in stress-reduction activities like yoga and meditation had lower cortisol levels and higher levels of estrogen and progesterone, indicating that lifestyle interventions may be effective in restoring hormonal balance.

Testosterone also has a role to play in women when it comes to mood especially dark thoughts and there is some (limited) evidence to-date that show that a lot of mental health issues really improve with testosterone It's not a quick fix - it can take months.

But, as we know, estrogen, in particular, plays a crucial role in managing the stress response, and both testosterone and estrogen are important for nerve health, both support the myelin sheath, our nerve protectors. This is important when it comes to the longer term impacts of alzheimers and dementia in women (Chatper 4).

As mentioned earlier, estrogen has been found to have a calming effect on the brain, because it influences the production and function of neurotransmitters like serotonin and dopamine, which are involved in mood regulation. When estrogen levels decline during menopause, this calming effect is reduced. Although covered in earlier chapters, a reminder that this is caused by too much cortisol - the stress hormone. Diet is introduced later and in the Chapter titled The Hormonal Diet.

Strategies to support anxiety, mood and depression

If you do start taking HRT, be patient. It can take time and the dose and type may need tweaking before you feel the beneficial effects.

Keep hydrated - the lack of fluids can cause anger, confusion, sadness, tension, and tiredness.

There is strong evidence that cognitive behavioral therapy (CBT) helps with anxiety, depression and other emotional challenges and although not specifically for menopause, it can help too.

People with depression and anxiety have lower levels of

Omega-3s. More high quality research is needed to know whether increasing consumption of fish or using omega-3 supplements, with or without other treatments, helps during peri-menopause and menopause but we know that there is an Omega-3 effect.

Stress and managing stress is incredibly important when it comes to not just your mental health but your overall health. And although this is important at any point in our life, when our hormone levels area falling and when they are out of balance we need to find the time and take measures to find ways of limiting stress and anxiety as much as we can. The ways that you can do this are covered in the chapter called The Hormonal Lifestyle and the following outlines what you can do.

Strategies for Managing Anxiety and Depression

- Mind-body techniques: Exploring relaxation techniques and practices that can help alleviate anxiety and reduce symptoms of depression.
- Deep breathing exercises
- Meditation and mindfulness
- Progressive muscle relaxation (often done as part of meditation)
- Expressive therapies: Discovering creative outlets that can aid in emotional expression and provide a sense of release and relief.
- Journaling and expressive writing
- Art therapy and creative expression
- Music therapy and listening to mood-enhancing music

Cultivating a Positive Menopausal Mindset

- Prioritise self-care activities
- Setting boundaries and saying no

- Practicing self-compassion and positive self-talk
- Cultivating gratitude and positivity: Incorporating gratitude practices and positive affirmations into your daily routine.
- Keeping a gratitude journal
- Practicing positive affirmations
- Surrounding yourself with positive influences and supportive people

Managing Stress and Building Resilience

- Stress management techniques: Exploring various strategies to manage and reduce stress during menopause.
- Time management and prioritization
- Stress-relieving exercises such as yoga or Tai Chi
- Setting realistic expectations and goals
- Building emotional resilience: Developing skills and habits that can help you bounce back from challenges and setbacks.
- Embracing flexibility and adaptability
- Nurturing a growth mindset
- Seeking support and building a strong support system

Interactive Exercise: Create a self-care plan tailored to your emotional well-being during menopause. Identify activities that bring you joy, relaxation, and emotional nourishment. Schedule regular self-care time and commit to engaging in those activities. Additionally, practice gratitude by writing down three things you are grateful for each day. Notice the positive impact this has on your emotional well-being.

FOUR

The Cognitive Challenge: Boosting Brain Power and Mood

Importantly, women face a disproportionate burden of Alzheimer's disease relative to men. Further, the neuropathological hallmarks of Alzheimer's are laid down beginning at midlife...

— Rebecca C. Thurston, Ph.D., University of Pittsburgh

Menopause can bring about changes in cognitive function, including memory lapses and difficulty concentrating. In this chapter, you'll discover strategies to boost your brain power and maintain cognitive health during and after menopause.

As we know, estradiol, a version of estrogen, is pretty much the star player during our reproductive years. It's like a supportive friend that helps with things like fine motor control and coordination. Ever misplaced your keys or forgot an important meeting? Estradiol is there to help, contributing to memory function and even boosting your mood.

Estrogen has been found to have a calming effect on the brain, because it influences the production and function of neurotransmitters like serotonin and dopamine, which are involved in mood regulation.

It also plays a role in the formation and maintenance of myelin - along with testosterone. Myelin is the protective coating around nerve fibers that helps transmit signals across the nervous system. Our nerve 'transmissions' let us know if we are anxious or not, it can mean low mood, brain fog, and it can make us (irrationally) upset and tearful and even cause pins and needles.

Acting as an inflammatory agent, estradiol can also help cool down your body when it's feeling a little heated or stressed. This helps decrease TH17 cells, a type of white blood cell that plays a key role in the immune system, and which can be quite the troublemakers, being linked with several autoimmune diseases such as multiple sclerosis (MS), psoriasis, and rheumatoid arthritis.

Myelin is the protective layer that surrounds nerve fibers. It is critical for the proper functioning of the nervous system because it enables efficient transmission of electrical signals along the nerve cells. In some autoimmune diseases, such as multiple sclerosis, the immune system mistakenly attacks the myelin sheath, disrupting the communication between nerve cells.

Research suggests that estradiol can enhance remyelination, which is the process of repairing damaged myelin, specifically, they help to protect the body against infections, as well as being involved in managing inflammatory responses and possibly these autoimmune diseases.

In other words, TH17 cells are part of the immune system that can, in some circumstances, contribute to the damage of myelin, but they are not a part of myelin itself.

So, estrogen or specifically estradiol, is good for nerve health which can help protect and grow the myelin sheath while also reducing inflammation. It works as a neurotransmitter and it can be very helpful in repairing any nerve damage.

Testosterone also has a significant role to play here. As well as helping to maintain muscle and bone strength and our libido (and clear up the "brain fog") it also helps the production of myelin.

This function makes it an integral part of our neuro-protective arsenal.

In the context of peri menopause, it can be difficult to attribute specific symptoms directly to changes in myelin or TH17 cells as these changes happen at a microscopic level within the body.

However, we can make educated guesses based on what we know about the functions of myelin and TH17 cells.

1. Cognitive changes: Myelin helps speed up signal transmission along nerves, including those in the brain. Changes in myelin could potentially contribute to cognitive changes, such as memory problems or "brain fog," that some women experience during peri menopause.

2. Fatigue: This could potentially be related to changes in nerve function. The immune system, including TH17 cells, also plays a role in managing the body's energy levels. Alterations in immune function could conceivably contribute to feelings of fatigue.

3. Muscle weakness or changes in muscle mass: Hormones like estradiol and testosterone play a role in maintaining muscle mass and strength. As levels of these hormones decrease during peri menopause, some women may experience a decrease in muscle mass or strength.

It's important to note that these symptoms can have multiple causes and are not solely due to changes in myelin or TH17 cells. In fact, other aspects of peri menopause, including changes in other hormones and general ageing processes, likely play a significant role.

Our memory is all about brain function and our nerves and this includes the energy, or food, that our nerve and brain cells need. Estrogen doesn't only care for our neurons, keeping them firing, and supporting new cell growth but it is also responsible for the glucose (or energy) the 'food' of our cells.

In the past 15-20 years, there has been a growing body of research investigating the intricate effects of menopause on the brain and identifying factors that help preserve memory function. Studies have shown that menopause can influence brain activity, including the generation, connectivity, and even death of brain cells. These processes specifically impact brain regions crucial for memory formation.

Because menopause leads to a decrease in glucose levels in brain cells, the primary energy source, as estrogen levels decline, the brain adapts to this hormonal shift by seeking alternative metabolic and energy sources to sustain itself. This can cause hot flashes and night sweats along with symptoms including anxiety, depression and brain fog.

Testosterone, once again has a role to play. It supports the strength of our nerves and our arteries - it keeps the blood flowing to our brain, protecting against memory loss. It means that testosterone keeps our minds sharp and clear.

So why does all this matter when it comes to menopause? According to Harvard Medical School, by 2050, 13.8 million people in the US are likely to have Alzheimer's disease, and two-thirds will be women. Now, from puberty up until mid-life women perform better than men on measures of verbal memory. We know that during menopause "brain fog" and forgetfulness is common, but on top of this, women's advantage for verbal memory performance has also been show to reduce, and often to below the level of men. It suggests a reversal. Menopause, which is caused by the lowering of our hormone levels, including estrogen and testosterone, does appear to have a direct impact on our cognitive function.

Why Menopause Puts Your Memory to the Test

I will list the research sources at the end of this chapter if you want to know more, because this is something that you may not already be aware of (all sources are at the end of the book) and it links many of the symptoms - it ties into cardiovascular health which links to hot flashes and night sweats, just as an example.

I will quote much of it below because this is so important for us all and I don't want to diminish what these researchers and doctors have found. But it also highlights the difference between chronological again and 'ovarian ageing' and why, men's health and women's health is so different - especially in terms of alzhiemer's, heart health and cognition.

As we touch on in the next chapter the vasomotor symptoms, hot flashes and night sweats and poor sleep are linked to greater risk of cardiovascular disease and because of the estrogen receptors that are present in regions of the brain associated with memory, such as the hippocampus, and this also effects our brain function.

These receptors influence the release and availability of neurotransmitters involved in memory formation and retrieval (and is linked to the nerve-protectors, myelin, sometimes called 'white matter'). This means that menopause can also have an impact on cognitive functions, including memory leading to memory lapses and difficulties in cognitive performance. But it can also impact your longer term susceptibility to alzhiemer's or dementia.

"A brain imaging study supported in part by NIA indicated differences in the brain's structure, connectivity, and energy process before, during, and after the menopausal transition. The study was led by Lisa Mosconi, Ph.D., director of the Weill Cornell Women's Brain Initiative. The findings showed that the brain changes were specific to menopausal ovarian aging rather than chronological aging."

"Our research team and others have demonstrated that estradiol directly relates to changes in memory performance and reorganization of our brain circuitry that regulates memory function."

The preliminary research showed that vasomotor symptoms were associated with poorer verbal memory (word encoding and word recognition) and altered brain activity during the memory task. "These symptoms, especially night sweats, were also associated with greater lesions in the brain called white matter hyperintensities."

Research from Harvard and a myriad of other organisations including the Cleveland Clinic also shows that estrogen contributes to language skills, attention, mood, memory, and other brain processes. The evidence seems conclusive: the decrease in estrogen (estradiol) that women experience at the time of the peri menopause and menopause, directly relates to changes in memory performance and the changes in our brain circuitry that regulates memory function.

Moreover, women with underlying medical conditions such as diabetes and hypertension face an increased risk of experiencing cognitive decline.

To understand this better, researchers are focusing the parallels between the brain and body and looking at energy production processes (metabolism) and the functioning of the vascular system, including blood pressure regulation.

I for one will be keeping up-to-date with this area of research because it will, at some point, shed more light on how menopause affects brain health and cognition, particularly memory, while also considering the interplay between hormonal changes, energy metabolism, heart health and vascular factors. We need much more information.

Hormone replacement is not always an option and other support and research needs to be identified, one of which might be glucose and other effects associated with estradiol regulation of the brain.

As you can see, while we might understand the underlying cause, the reasons why our brains are effected in the way that they are don't all appear to be due to the same estrogen effect, and it's fair to say that we don't yet fully know what the range of changes they have on our different body systems and organs which declining estrogen and other hormones cause. What we do know is that it can, and in many cases, that it does. So much so that even doctors who specialise in this field take HRT to protect against alzhiemer's (and osteoporosis) in later life.

A word of caution however, it depends when you begin HRT. Current evidence suggests that while starting hormone replacement in peri-menopause or early menopause can have positive effects on brain activity and memory function, beginning it in late menopause may have adverse effects and actually increase the risk of disorders like Alzheimer's. It's one very good reason to explore this sooner rather than later and to consider some kind of hormone replacement strategy.

It's important to note that these cognitive changes are typically subtle and do vary from woman to woman. Some women may notice mild forgetfulness or difficulty concentrating, while others may not experience any significant impact.

What can women do to maintain brain health?

According to Harvard Health, the three pillars for maintaining memory include physical, cognitive 'effortful' activity which have a direct beneficial effects on the brain, along with social contact. Although not always in the top 3, sleep is also vital, particularly for brain health.

Physical activity includes aerobic and weight bearing exercises and we talk about these in the Hormone Lifestyle later in the book.

The Mediterranean diet and other nutrients like omega-3 fatty are important in terms of diet and memory function, and as we know, a good diet helps with many of the problems that we experience. This, too, is covered throughout the book as well as in the chapter called The Hormonal Diet.

Don't forget that Soy isoflavones have been found to slightly improve memory in postmenopausal women but more studies are needed in women in peri menopause. It was not helpful for other aspects of cognition, such as attention and executive function.

How to Sharpen Your Mind and Focus

- Engaging your brain: Exploring activities and exercises that can help stimulate your brain, improve memory, and enhance cognitive function.
- Brain-training exercises and puzzles
- Learning new skills or languages
- Reading and staying mentally active
- Managing stress for better cognitive health: Understanding the connection between stress and cognitive function and implementing stress management techniques.
- Relaxation techniques, such as deep breathing and meditation
- Time management and prioritization
- Seeking support and utilizing coping strategies

Habits for Maintaining Cognitive Health

- Getting quality sleep: Recognizing the importance of sleep in memory and cognitive function and implementing strategies for better sleep hygiene.
- Establishing a consistent sleep schedule
- Creating a relaxing bedtime routine
- Creating a sleep-friendly environment

- Regular Exercise including Aerobic exercises and Strength training

Nutrition for Brain Power

- Omega-3 fatty acids and their sources
- Antioxidant-rich fruits and vegetables
- Foods high in vitamins B6 and B12
- Hydration - don't forget to drink lots of water

Interactive Exercises:

Engage in brain-training exercises and puzzles, such as crosswords or Sudoku, for 15 minutes each day (my personal favorite is Wordle!) . Track your progress and note any improvements in memory, focus, or problem-solving abilities. Additionally, incorporate relaxation techniques, such as deep breathing or meditation, into your daily routine to reduce stress and enhance cognitive function.

Start a mood journal to track your emotions and identify patterns in your mood swings. Note any triggers, symptoms, and the duration of your mood swings. This exercise will help you gain insight into your emotional patterns and provide valuable information for managing your mood swings effectively.

Chapter Resources

1. *Women's Brain Initiative:* https://neurology.weill.cornell. edu/research/womens-brain-initiative
2. *Impact of Sex and Menopausal Status on Episodic Memory Circuitry in Early Midlife*: https://pubmed.ncbi.nlm.nih. gov/27683911/

3. *Sex differences in episodic memory in early midlife:* Impact of reproductive aging https://www.ncbi.nlm.nih.gov/pmc/articles/PMC5365356/

4. *Impact of BDNF and sex on maintaining intact memory function in early midlife*: https://pubmed.ncbi.nlm.nih.gov/31948671/

5. *Human Brain Mapping:* https://www.ncbi.nlm.nih.gov/pmc/articles/PMC6365200/

6. *Objective hot flashes are negatively related to verbal memory performance in midlife women:* https://pubmed.ncbi.nlm.nih.gov/18562950/

7. *Oophorectomy, menopause, estrogen treatment, and cognitive aging: clinical evidence for a window of opportunity*: https://pubmed.ncbi.nlm.nih.gov/20965156/

FIVE

Hot Flashes and Night Sweats: The Uninvited Guests

The hormonal effects on vasomotor symptoms (VMS) can often begin early in peri menopause, and if they do, then your hot flashes and hight sweats can last as long as 10 years. If the symptoms start after your last period then they shouldn't last as long.

They are experienced by over 70% of women and, for a third of women, they are frequent or severe. At one time they were thought to only last for a few years but more recent data (2023) indicates that frequent or moderate-severe VMS lasts on average 7–10 years and for many women, much longer.

Hot flashes and night sweats (or VMS for the purposes on understanding the research) are not insignificant to women's health.

A report in 2023 by the American Academy of Neurology highlights the "burgeoning body of data (that) links them to physical health" and goes on to say that multiple studies have found more frequent VMS is associated with higher cardiovascular disease (CVD) risk.

The same research paper, that includes one of the largest

studies to-date, concludes that there is evidence that it might be explained by greater white matter (nerves and myelin) hyperintensity volume (WMHV). It links hot flashes and night sweats to cardiovascular health as well as memory decline including alzheimer's.

Hot flashes and night sweats are the most common and earliest symptoms of peri menopause and the one that has a significant effect on day-to-day life for women.

Hot flashes can have a dramatic effect of work as the rising tide of heat surges across the body, reddening our faces and having us dash for a door or try to hide from colleagues or avoid meetings. This is where much better workplace understanding is needed. While colleagues may mean well, asking if 'you are alright' or 'you look unwell, maybe you need to go home' means that this natural life process feels like an illness or something to 'hide'. It shouldn't be, nor should it be the butt of jokes.

I was with my hair dresser just yesterday and she was talking about how she used to suddenly ask her client if a coffee was needed so that she could dash to the kitchen, or she would helpfully move the hairdryer around and comment how hot it was, eventually leaving the door the salon open until it got too uncomfortable for her clients. She found it so disruptive to her business life that she went on HRT which solved her problem.

Because hot flashes and flushes are so 'public' and 'embarrassing' - what better an indicator of age and of feeling 'old' than a bright red face and over-heating - this is often the main reason that women seek out solutions, often HRT or other forms of hormone replacement.

Night sweats keep us up at night, as we try to cool down or change our bedding, sometimes more than once. I know of more than one women who stopped going for any over-night stays, including hotels and guesthouses and certainly never with friends. This was not easy because she had to travel for work too. But it is the lack of sleep that can have the biggest impact. It multiplies existing feelings of lethargy and exhaustion which does nothing to support our already fragile mental health.

Hot flashes and nights sweats: what's going on

For the purposes of this chapter, we will look at hot flashes and night sweats which have their root in our hypothalamus, which, as we know, is the region of the brain that is responsible for regulating body temperature. It receives signals from various hormones, including estrogen and progesterone, and during menopause, as estrogen levels decline, the hypothalamus becomes more sensitive to even slight changes in hormone levels.

In a bid to cool things down, it triggers mechanisms like sweating and widening of the blood vessels (vasodilation). This results in the hot flush as well as the night sweat. As the hypothalamus perceives a rise in body temperature, it starts a cascade of events to cool the body down. Blood vessels in the skin dilate, allowing more blood to flow to the surface, and perspiration increases to enhance evaporative cooling. This sudden dilation and constriction of blood vessels, along with the accompanying sweating, result in the characteristic hot flashes and night sweats.

But it doesn't stop there. From an earlier chapter we know that menopause can also have an impact on cognitive functions, including memory. Estrogen plays a crucial role in maintaining brain health and cognitive processes. As estrogen levels decline, certain areas of the brain involved in memory and cognitive function may experience changes.

There are other factors at play including noradrenaline (or norepinephrine), also managed by the hypothalamus which, as well as temperature, affects mood and attention, as well as Serotonin - both examples of neurotransmitters that play a role in controlling body temperature. Both are impacted by declining estrogen.

Hot flashes, also known as hot flushes, are sudden feelings of warmth spreading over the body, but they are particularly noticeable on the face and upper body. Accompanying these sensations might be red, patchy skin (like a 'flush'), palpitations, or sweating.

Night sweats, although similar, also lead to disruptive sleep and are often accompanied by heavy sweating.

We know that hormones like melatonin and cortisol also play roles in sleep regulation, and with night sweats both of these play a part - caused again by the hypothalamus not only believing that the body is over-heating but also triggering cortisol and melatonin - two sleep disrupters.

What might cool you down

While hormonal changes are at the core, lifestyle factors can make things worse. Certain triggers like caffeine, alcohol, spicy foods, stress, and smoking can increase their frequency and severity by stimulating the nervous system or affecting blood vessels, prompting those temperature fluctuations.

Numerous research efforts have focused on the impact of soy-based products - including foods, supplements, and powders.

Soy contains three phytoestrogens or plant-based estrogen called "isoflavones" (genistein and daidzein). Our gut bacteria changes daidzein into a chemical called equol and it is this that acts like a weak estrogen. Because not all women can make equol (only 20% of US women) equol is often taken as a supplement.

Equol has been found in studies to potentially reduce both the frequency and intensity of daytime hot flashes, provided it is taken in sufficient amounts (a total of 100-200mg per day) and it might also offer some relief from night sweats.

Soy-based foods include soy sauce, tofu, soy milk, soy yogurt, edamame (immature soybeans), miso, and tempeh, but, overall, studies suggest that soy isoflavones may relieve hot flashes but that they don't appear to relieve night sweats (unlike, oddly, the soy-based equol).

A recent study has also found that sage can help control hot flashes, night sweats, and other symptoms in postmenopausal women. In this double-blind randomised controlled trial, 66 post-menopausal women took either a 100 mg sage tablet or placebo three times a day for three months. The results found that the women who took sage experienced significant decreases in night sweats and hot flashes at ten weeks and 12 weeks and reported improvements in sleep, mood, anxiety levels, sex drive, forgetful-ness, and more. I happen to love sage, and it's well worth a try.

How to manage the symptoms

While the science behind vasomotor symptoms and cognitive changes during menopause is complex and still the subject of much research, there are strategies that can help manage these symptoms.

Hormone replacement therapy (HRT) can be effective by supplementing the declining estrogen, progesterone and testos-terone levels. You will need to work with your healthcare provider to find the right dosage, frequency, along with the best applica-tion for you (pill, patch, gel and so on). My hairdresser mentioned above started with patches, eventually changing to pills.

In addition to medical interventions, lifestyle changes can also make a difference. Regular exercise, a balanced diet, stress reduc-tion techniques, and maintaining a healthy sleep routine can contribute to overall well-being during menopause.

Hormone Replacement Therapy (HRT) is often the first port of call in managing hot flushes and night sweats. By replacing the declining estrogen, HRT can help to stabilize the body's thermostat and help with both daytime flushes and flashes as well as night sweats. Progesterone helps relieve some hot flashes and night sweats, but does not eliminate them. It may also help with sleep problems.

Non-Hormonal Medications: There are also non-hormonal prescription options that can be effective. Some antidepressants, for instance, have been shown to alleviate hot flushes, possibly due to their effect on the serotonin system (SSRIs). Other medications, like certain anti-seizure drugs and blood pressure medications, can also help reduce hot flushes.

Other Natural Remedies and Supplements: Some people find relief with natural remedies such as black cohosh, red clover, and, as discussed, soy. The best ones are probably Soy and Red Clover (great as a tea). Additionally, a study published in the journal, Menopause, found that black cohosh improved hot flashes. Be careful with Black Cohosh because it can damage your liver so avoid this if you have any liver problems. Sage is also for good for night sweats but may not help with hot flashes.

Dietary Adjustments: Certain triggers can increase the frequency and severity of hot flushes and night sweats. These include spicy foods, caffeine, and alcohol. Reducing intake of these triggers can help keep your internal thermostat in check.

Smoking Cessation: Smoking can increase the frequency and severity of hot flushes, so if you're a smoker, consider seeking help to quit.

Stay Cool: Keep your environment cool, especially at night. Consider using a fan or an air conditioner, dressing in layers so you can adjust your clothing as needed and using cooling pillows or sheets at night. Wear natural fibres like cotton and drink lots of water.

Regular Exercise: Regular physical activity can help regulate hormonal balance, reduce stress, and improve sleep. Find a type of exercise that you enjoy and incorporate it into your daily routine.

Stress Management: Techniques like mindfulness, yoga,

meditation, and deep-breathing exercises can help manage stress, which can, in turn, help reduce hot flushes and night sweats.

Bedtime Routine: Establish a regular sleep schedule. Create a relaxing bedtime routine, like reading or listening to soothing music.

Chapter resources

- *Menopausal Vasomotor Symptoms and White Matter Hyperintensities in Midlife Women* https://www.ncbi.nlm.nih.gov/pmc/articles/PMC9841446/
- *Carotid intima media thickness and white matter hyperintensity volume among midlife women* https://pubmed.ncbi.nlm.nih.gov/36722746/
- *The effect of Salvia officinalis extract on symptoms of flushing, night sweat, sleep disorders,* and score of forgetfulness in postmenopausal women. J Family Med Prim Care. February 2020;9(2):1086-1092. doi: 10.4103/jfmpc.jfmpc_913_19.

SIX

Tackling Tiredness: Boosting Your Energy

F atigue and lack of energy are common symptoms of menopause, but there are practical steps you can take to boost your energy levels and combat tiredness during this phase of life.

Sleep is an incredibly important part of health that is very often overlooked. It effects a myriad of health issue effecting stress levels and mental well-being. But as we navigate the menopause, sleep, that once loyal friend, can often turn elusive. The Sandman's visits seem fewer and further between, replaced instead by wakeful nights and restless hours spent watching the mocking hands of the clock.

In the quiet of the night, many women in the throes of menopause find themselves wide-eyed, wrestling with discomforts like hot flashes, night sweats, anxiety, and an unpredictable internal thermostat. It's like trying to sleep on an ever-changing canvas of discomfort, from an inferno one moment to an ice field the next.

Think about it. Is there anything more disorienting than watching the day break while struggling to silence the whirlwind of thoughts in your head? How many of us have sat helplessly as exhaustion seeped into our bones, even as our minds buzzed like overcharged circuits? Or tried to function on an energy level comparable to a drained smartphone, moving through the day in a state of semi-conscious fatigue?

Let's add to that the cascade of physiological changes that menopause triggers. The fluctuating hormones can disturb the body's internal clock, interrupting the usual rhythm of sleep. And there's also a decrease in the production of melatonin, the sleep hormone. Combined, they create the perfect storm for sleep disturbances.

But do we really understand the full impact of these sleepless nights? Apart from the obvious fatigue and exhaustion, poor sleep can exacerbate mood swings, trigger weight gain, compromise immune function, and even impair memory. Each restless night chips away not just at our energy, but our overall health and quality of life.

Sleep should not be a luxury or an elusive dream. It is a pillar of health, as critical as diet and exercise, and even more crucial during the transformative years of menopause.

Understanding Sleep and Its Role in Our Health

Sleep, it turns out, is far more complex and critical than we often give it credit for. It involves a range of biological processes, conducted by our body's internal clock or circadian rhythm. This 24-hour internal clock regulates not only our sleep-wake cycle but also influences hormone production, cell regeneration, and various other physiological processes.

While we sleep, our bodies are not simply resting but are actively working to repair cells, strengthen the immune system, consolidate memories, and regulate hormones, including those responsible for appetite and metabolism. Each of these processes is crucial to our overall health, and disturbances in sleep can lead to a wide range of health problems - from increased vulnerability to illnesses, emotional disturbances, cognitive impairment, to even chronic conditions like heart disease and diabetes.

The Science of Menopause and Sleep

So, how does menopause affect this critical process?

The decline in levels of estrogen and progesterone can directly impact sleep. For instance, progesterone has sleep-promoting effects and a decline in its levels can contribute to sleep disturbances.

Meanwhile, decreasing estrogen levels can lead to hot flashes - sudden feelings of heat all over the body - and night sweats, both of which can cause nighttime awakenings and disrupted sleep. Similarly, changes in estrogen levels can cause mood swings and increase anxiety, which in turn can lead to insomnia.

The Connection Between Sleep and Other Menopausal Symptoms

And it's not just the hormone changes. Lack of sleep can further exacerbate other menopausal symptoms. As we saw in an earlier chapter, sleep deprivation can worsen hot flashes and night sweats, leading to a vicious cycle of disturbed sleep. Similarly, poor sleep can amplify mood swings, irritability, and anxiety, and even contribute to memory problems.

Lack of sleep also takes a toll on our metabolic functions. It affects the way our bodies store fat and regulate blood sugar levels, leading to weight gain and increasing the risk of metabolic disorders. This is particularly relevant to menopausal women, who are already at a higher risk of gaining weight due to hormonal changes.

Sleep and why it leads to weight-gain

Sleep, it turns out, is critical for hormonal balance. During sleep, your body produces and releases important hormones like growth hormone and melatonin, which play vital roles in various bodily functions. When you don't get enough sleep or experience poor-quality sleep, your hormonal balance can be thrown off.

According to a study by the National Sleep Foundation, lack of sleep can disrupt the balance of hormones in the body. Specifically, the hormones responsible for regulating appetite, ghrelin, and leptin, are affected by sleep deprivation. Ghrelin is the hormone that signals hunger to the brain, while leptin is the hormone that signals fullness. When you don't get enough sleep, ghrelin levels increase, making you hungrier, while leptin levels decrease, making it harder for you to feel satisfied after eating.

Another study published in the Journal of Clinical Endocrinology & Metabolism found that after just one week of sleep deprivation, as well as lower leptin levels and higher levels of ghrelin, the study found that sleep deprivation can also affect insulin sensitivity (leading to higher blood sugar levels and an increased risk of developing type 2 diabetes).

It all means that these disruptions in hormone balance can lead to overeating, weight gain, and increased risk for conditions like type 2 diabetes and heart disease. Sleep deprivation can also increase cortisol levels, the stress hormone, contributing to inflammation, mood disorders, and other health issues.

In short, getting enough sleep is essential for maintaining hormonal balance and overall health. The National Sleep Foundation recommends adults aim for 7-9 hours of sleep each night to support optimal health and well-being.

Melatonin

Melatonin is a hormone produced by the pineal gland that regulates sleep-wake cycles. It is often called the "sleep hormone" because it helps you fall asleep and stay asleep.

There are specialised light receiving cells in your retinas that tell your brain to stop making the sleep hormone melatonin and light also stimulates production of the hormone cortisol, to help get your brain fired up for the day. A light early morning walk will usually help you fall asleep more quickly at night too.

Try and get at least 15 to 30 minutes outside in the morning and then again between 1-3pm when the body produces another brief spike of sleep hormone.

If this isn't possible, position yourself facing a window or failing that, add some more indoor light via lamps near to your face.

But, whatever you do, try to get lots of sun and light to boost your melatonin. It boosts your mood too.

Mindfulness and Cognitive Behavioral Therapy

A critical first step towards better sleep during menopause is cultivating a mindful approach. This involves acknowledging and understanding your sleep patterns and disturbances without judgment or frustration.

Mindfulness practices such as meditation and controlled breathing exercises can help manage the stress and anxiety associated with menopause, which can help with relaxation and better sleep. These practices also help in training your mind to disconnect from the buzzing thoughts and worries that often accompany the silent hours of the night.

Cognitive Behavioral Therapy for Insomnia (CBT-I) is another effective approach for improving sleep. This therapy helps to challenge and change thought patterns that lead to sleep anxiety, replacing them with healthier beliefs and attitudes about sleep. Through CBT-I, women can learn to establish a regular sleep schedule, optimize their sleep environment, and practice relaxation techniques that can improve both sleep quality and duration.

The Role of Nutrition and Exercise

Diet and physical activity can also play a significant role in managing menopausal symptoms and promoting better sleep. Consuming a balanced diet rich in fruits, vegetables, lean proteins, and complex carbohydrates can help maintain stable blood sugar levels and prevent nighttime hunger pangs.

Certain foods like cherries, nuts, and dairy products contain natural sources of melatonin and can help enhance sleep. Limiting caffeine and alcohol, especially close to bedtime, can also promote better sleep as these substances can interfere with your sleep cycle.

Regular physical activity, meanwhile, has been shown to reduce hot flashes, improve mood, and promote better sleep. Even light activities, like a daily walk or yoga, can make a significant difference.

Creating a Sleep-Friendly Environment

Your sleep environment also plays a crucial role in your sleep quality. A cool, dark, and quiet room can help manage hot flashes and prevent sleep disturbances. Using breathable sheets, wearing light sleepwear, and even considering a cooling pillow can make a world of difference.

Furthermore, establishing a sleep routine that signals to your body that it's time to sleep can help reinforce your body's natural sleep-wake cycle. This can include a relaxing pre-sleep ritual, like reading a book, listening to soft music, or taking a warm bath.

While lifestyle modifications and self-care strategies can significantly improve sleep, it's important to seek medical advice when these disturbances persist or severely impact your quality of life. Healthcare providers can explore other treatment options, such as hormone replacement therapy (HRT), low-dose antidepressants, or other medications that can manage hot flashes and improve sleep.

Remember, while menopause and aging is a natural phase of life, struggling with sleep does not have to be.

If you can't or don't want to explore HRT, or other medications, then there are lots of Herbal remedies that have been used for centuries to treat a wide range of ailments, including sleep problems associated with menopause.

Here are a few that have shown some promise:

Ashwagandha root has been found to reduce stress leading to better sleep and lower blood cortisol levels. Like any herb, don't overuse it, check the amount and frequency of use.

Black Cohosh: This plant has been used for generations to help alleviate symptoms of menopause, including hot flashes and night sweats that can disrupt sleep. Some research has suggested it may have estrogen-like effects in the body, but its full mechanisms aren't fully understood. Once again, don't use this herb if you have any liver problems and don't overuse.

Valerian Root: Valerian is a herb that has been used for centuries as a remedy for various ailments, including insomnia. Some studies suggest that it may help to improve sleep quality and reduce the time it takes to fall asleep.

Chamomile: Chamomile tea is often recommended as a sleep aid due to its calming effects. It can also help with digestion, which might be helpful if stomach upset is contributing to sleep problems.

Lavender: The scent of lavender is known to have a calming effect and has been used to improve sleep quality. It can be used in various ways, such as in a diffuser, in bath products, or as an essential oil.

Lemon Balm: Lemon balm, a member of the mint family, is often used to reduce stress and anxiety, improve sleep, and ease discomfort from indigestion (including bloating and gas). It's often combined with other calming herbs like valerian and chamomile in sleep-promoting tea blends.

Passionflower: Traditionally used to treat anxiety and insomnia, passionflower can help to promote sleep. It can be consumed as a tea, tincture, or in capsule form.

Red Clover: Red clover is rich in isoflavones, plant compounds that have estrogen-like effects in the body. There is some evidence to back this up and many women find it helpful for reducing hot flashes and night sweats.

Interactive Exercise: Energy-boosting plan

Create a personalized energy-boosting plan by identifying your energy drains and implementing strategies to counteract them. Consider your daily routines, stressors, and lifestyle choices. Experiment with different techniques and habits to find what works best for you in increasing your energy levels.

SEVEN

The Aura and The Migraine

A migraine is a type of headache characterized by a moderate to severe throbbing pain, typically affecting one side of the head. Accompanying symptoms often include nausea, vomiting, and an increased sensitivity to light and sound. The intensity of the pain is usually debilitating enough to interfere with daily activities and can persist from four to 72 hours.

You may, or many not know this, but migraines can often come with a phase known as an 'aura'. This can include visual disturbances such as seeing spots, flashing lights, or zigzag lines, along with vertigo, dizziness, and sensations of numbness or tingling. It can begin anywhere from a few minutes to an hour before the headache.

While the majority of people experience migraines without an aura, those who do experience it understandably find that it serves as a warning of the impending headache. Interestingly, in some cases referred to as 'silent migraines,' individuals experience aura symptoms but no ensuing headache.

Migraines have a notable connection with hormones, particularly in women who are 2-3 times more likely to suffer from migraines than men. These are once again triggered by fluctuating hormone levels, especially dips in estrogen, progesterone and histamine.

This typically occurs a day or two before menstruation begins or during the hormone-free week (for those on combined oral contraceptive pills (COCP) or Hormone Replacement Therapy). If menopause is induced surgically, such as through a hysterectomy, migraines may initially become more frequent, before eventually subsiding.

After menopause, the frequency of migraines generally decreases as the hormonal fluctuations stabilise, but this process may take years or even decades for some women.

If you are using HRT, and aiming to also manage your migraine, it's advised to use a transdermal application using the estrogen patch, gel, or spray continuously, without any interruptions. This steady use will mean the you receive a constant delivery of the hormone directly into your bloodstream, avoiding sudden fluctuations in estrogen levels which can trigger a migraine.

It's generally considered good practice to start with a low dosage of transdermal estrogen and then slowly escalate the dosage if your symptoms aren't showing signs of improvement.

It's important to note that not all migraines are hormone-related, so some women may continue to experience migraines well after menopause, even when using hormonal treatments.

EIGHT

Hair, Skin & Collagen

C hanges to the skin and hair are pretty common during peri menopause and menopause and, once again, this is due to the decline in progesterone and estrogen.

In fact, nearly half of women visiting a menopause clinic report experiencing skin issues as a result of menopause. Let's walk through some of the common skin problems and what you can do to ease them.

Skin and Hair

Does your skin feel itchy and dry? That's quite common around menopause. Estrogen helps keep our skin hydrated by helping it produce ceramides, natural hyaluronic acid, and sebum. When these elements reduce, your skin can dry out making it feel 'saggy'.

So, what can you do about it? Ditch soaps that bubble or foam; they tend to strip the natural oils from your skin. Use a gentle, non-foaming cleanser instead. If that doesn't do the trick, try a moisturising lotion as a soap substitute. Make it a habit to moisturise your skin twice daily, especially after a bath or shower. You might want to consider lighter moisturisers for the day and something a bit richer for the night. If you're still itching, it's worth discussing with your doctor as other factors like iron deficiency or thyroid disturbance could be at play.

Experiencing redness and flushing? That's another symptom of menopause. It could also be rosacea, where blood vessels in the skin become overly reactive. You can manage these symptoms by reducing your alcohol and caffeine intake, avoiding spicy foods, and protecting your skin from sun exposure. In some cases, you might need creams or laser treatments to help shrink blood vessels in the skin.

And let's not forget those pesky spots and acne. They can be distressing, particularly during menopause. If you're dealing with these, make sure your makeup and sun protection products are all noncomedogenic (meaning, they won't aggravate acne). A mild cleanser with salicylic acid can help unclog pores, and skincare ingredients like retinol and niacinamide may help keep breakouts at bay.

Facial hair growth can be a nuisance, too. You might notice thick hairs developing on the upper lip, chin, cheeks, and jawline. You can manage this with hair removal methods such as plucking, waxing, threading, shaving, and depilatory creams. Electrolysis and laser hair removal can offer a more permanent solution.

Signs of sun damage, like an uneven skin tone, dull skin, and sunspots, can become more visible around menopause. To prevent further damage, wear high-factor SPF sunscreen (like Factor 50), reapply it every two hours when you're in the sun, and wear a wide-brimmed hat and long sleeves whenever possible.

When it comes to hair, many women start to notice that their hair becomes thinner, drier, and more prone to breakage.

This is because, when estrogen levels drop, hair might spend less time in the growth phase and more time in the shedding phase and it is this that results in hair loss or thinning. On top of this, lower estrogen levels can lead to a decrease in sebum production, which is the oil that, as well as being good for your skin, naturally moisturises your scalp and hair. This can make your hair feel drier and more brittle.

For skin, it is also the lack of estrogen that makes it thinner, drier and less elastic leading to wrinkles and sagging. And, as above, it can also mean that your skin loses its ability to retain moisture which can cause dryness and itching while oil production is also reduced which makes it dryer and more prone to sensitivity.

Estrogen is responsible for collagen and sebum production and it is this that keeps your hair and skin healthy.

While the hypothalamic-pituitary-gonadal (HPG) axis plays an important role in regulating estrogen production, other systems and cells in the body are responsible for managing collagen and sebum levels.

Collagen is a protein that forms the building blocks of our skin which our bodies naturally produce through cells called fibroblasts. While both osteoblasts and fibroblasts produce collagen, they have distinct roles and functions in the body, and the collagen they produce serves different purposes. At, and 'after' menopause, collagen reduces as about 2% a year - unless you can help to support it with estrogen.

The collagen produced by fibroblasts helps provide structural support, strength, and flexibility to various tissues, such as skin, tendons, and ligaments. It is like a scaffold, supporting the skin and keeping it looking youthful and plump.

Sebum is an oily substance produced by sebaceous glands, which are located in the skin's dermis layer. Sebum plays a crucial role in maintaining skin and hair health by providing a natural barrier that keeps moisture in and helps protect our skin and hair from damage.

Estrogen has a stimulating effect on both collagen and sebum production, so when estrogen levels decline during menopause, these processes can be affected.

For collagen, lower estrogen levels can result in a decrease in the activity of fibroblasts, and this reduction in collagen production leads to a loss of skin elasticity and firmness, making the skin more prone to wrinkles and sagging.

As for sebum, its production is influenced by various hormones, including androgens (such as testosterone) and estrogens (like estradiol) and although sebum production is mainly regulated by androgens, estradiol influences sebum production by regulating the activity of androgen receptors and sebaceous glands.

It means that estrogen helps regulate the sebaceous glands that produce this essential oil. When estrogen levels drop, these glands become less active, leading to a reduction in sebum production. This can cause the skin and hair to become drier, more sensitive, and less protected against environmental factors.

Just like our skin, our vagina also suffers from the same effects with a thinning uterine wall, and less elasticity and firmness - and this contributes to vaginal pain - which can often appear well into your sixties.

Remedies

Collagen is a protein that is primarily made from chains of amino acids, I mention this because it helps understand what to look out for when you are thinking about a way to support or replace collagen loss.

Peptide-based collagen supplements, also known as hydrolyzed collagen or collagen peptides, are made from collagen proteins that have been broken down into smaller, more easily absorbed parts and the hydrolyzation process makes the collagen more bioavailable, allowing it to be more easily absorbed and used by the body.

There are several types of these collagen supplements available, including bovine (cow), porcine (pig), and marine (fish) collagen. Marine collagen is derived from fish skin and scales and this is often recommended due to its high bioavailability and potential to be more easily absorbed by the body - it is also a more sustainable option compared to bovine and porcine collagen sources.

More than this, this Type I collagen is the most similar to the collagen found in our bodies.

When you consume marine collagen, you provide your body with the building blocks it needs to stimulate collagen production in the deeper layers of the skin. This level of support is beyond the reach of traditional topical serums and lotions, which are limited in their ability to penetrate the skin's surface. In essence, Marine collagen provides the amino acids that contribute to the formation of new collagen, elastin, and other essential skin proteins.

For this reason, marine collagen is a good option as a way to improve skin heath and deal with some of your wrinkles. But it's not only the skin that this type of collagen is good for.

- Joint health: Marine collagen contains type I collagen, which is a primary component of joint cartilage. It means that this type of collagen can help maintain joint health.
- Hair and nail health: As well as supporting the skin it provides amino acids that support the health and growth of hair and nails, potentially leading to stronger, more resilient nails (and thicker, healthier hair).
- Muscle mass: Collagen is involved in muscle tissue repair and growth and this means that using supplements may help to improved muscle mass and

strength, especially when combined with resistance training.

- Gut health: Because collagen contains amino acids such as glycine, proline, and glutamine, which can support gut health by promoting the growth and repair of the intestinal lining it might help with symptoms of conditions such as leaky gut syndrome and inflammatory bowel disease (IBD).
- Heart health: Collagen is essential for maintaining the structure and function of blood vessels and it is believed to improve cardiovascular health by promoting blood vessel elasticity and reducing arterial stiffness.

There are lots of these products on the market and the optimal dosage of marine collagen supplements can vary depending on factors such as individual needs, the specific product, and the desired health benefits. Generally, a daily dosage of 5 to 10 grams of hydrolyzed marine collagen is considered a safe and effective starting point for most people. Some studies have used dosages up to 20 grams per day.

Marine collagen supplements mighty contain additional ingredients, such as Vitamin C which can help improve their effectiveness, Hyaluronic acid which is a naturally occurring substance which helps retain moisture in the skin and joints. Marine collagen supplements, especially in powder form, don't taste particularly great but it can contain natural or artificial flavorings and sweeteners. Otherwise try adding to a herbal tea to mask the taste.

When selecting a marine collagen supplement, it's essential to read the label carefully to understand the ingredients and their percentages. Look for a product with a high concentration of hydrolyzed marine collagen.

There are lots to choose from. Davina McCall, who kicked-off the nationwide awareness of menopause in the UK, uses Ancient + Brave (and reportedly she used bovine collagen). Bovine collagen is a good option if you have shellfish or fish allergies or are looking to support gut health as a priority.

Herbal and Plant Remedies

Collagen is a protein made up of amino acids, such as glycine, proline, hydroxyproline, and others. While no plant or herb contains collagen itself some plants contain amino acids or other compounds that can help.

Because they don't contain the exact amino acid profile found in collagen itself, you can help boost collagen production by including other nutrients such as vitamin C and minerals like copper and zinc, all of which play a role in collagen synthesis. This might include vitamin C-rich fruits and vegetables like citrus fruits, strawberries, kiwi, bell peppers, and leafy greens.

Here are a few ideas and all of these contain amino acids:

Once again we have **Soy**, and products, such as tofu, tempeh, and edamame (immature soybeans), all of which are rich in amino acids and contains genistein, which can help boost collagen production by helping support estrogen-like actions.

All the **legumes**, beans, lentils, and chickpeas are excellent sources of plant-based protein and contain a variety of amino acids which also have estrogen-like properties. Both Soy and legumes are often referred to as phytoestrogens - plant-based compounds that behave like estrogen in the body.

The blue-green algae, **Sprulina**, is a complete protein source, containing all essential amino acids required for collagen synthesis and its not too difficult to buy as a powder in the grocery store or supermarket.

Chia **seeds**, flaxseeds, and pumpkin seeds are also rich in amino acids, including lysine, which is also essential for collagen production.

Almonds, walnuts, and peanuts are not only good sources of amino acids but they have other nutrients that can support collagen synthesis.

Dark **leafy greens** including spinach and kale s are rich source of amino acids and antioxidants, which all help collagen production and can protect it from damage.

Quinoa, brown rice, and other whole grains are also all good sources of amino acids, including the ones needed for collagen production.

Red Clover is rich in phytoestrogens and encourages detoxification and promotes healthy skin by supporting the lymphatic functions. It is particularly good at supporting the body during during menopause.

In summary, while these plant-based phytoestrogens can help support collagen production, because they don't contain the exact amino acid profile found in collagen itself, you will need to include other nutrients such as vitamin C and minerals like copper and zinc, all of which play a role in collagen production.

NINE

The Bone Density Dilemma: Staying Strong and Sturdy

Hip pain, back pain, and fractures are some of the most common symptoms of osteoporosis. According to the National Osteoporosis Foundation, about 54 million Americans have osteoporosis or low bone mass, which puts them at increased risk for fractures. In fact, women can lose up to 20% of their bone density in the 5-7 years after menopause. Women over 50 are at an increased risk for osteoporotic fractures, particularly in the spine, hip, and wrist.

In addition to the physical risks, osteoporosis can also have emotional and social consequences. Fear of falling or fracturing bones can lead to social isolation and decreased quality of life.

Our skeleton is like a storehouse for two important minerals, calcium and phosphorus, which our body needs to work properly. These minerals are used by all the organs in our body, especially our nerves and muscles. To make sure we always have enough, our body has a complicated system of hormones that help to regulate the amount of these minerals.

This means that bones have to do two things at the same time: they need to be strong and sturdy to support our weight, but they also need to give up calcium and phosphorus when other parts of the body need it like our intestines and kidneys.

Bones are living tissue that constantly change throughout our lives. Our bone mass increases during childhood and adolescence, it reaches its peak in our late 20s or early 30s, and then begins to decline. As we will see, our bodies are designed to break down old bone and rebuild new bone and this process is regulated by hormones like estrogen, progesterone, and testosterone. There are other hormones involved such as parathyroid hormone (**PTH**) and Calcitonin but to keep things simple we will focus on the role of estrogen and progesterone.

This is the reason women start to lose bone mass at a faster rate than men do after the age of 50 and why they are more likely than men to have osteoporosis - as women age, our hormone levels naturally decline, and this can affect the body's ability to build new bone and maintain bone strength.

We will lose around 10% of our bone mass over the first 5 years of menopause. Other bone-related conditions include osteopenia, arthritis, and joint pain.

Once again, the earlier you apply some kind of hormone support the better the chance you have of minimising the effects of these conditions.

Bone Composition - A Closer Look at the Building Blocks

Bones are complex structures composed of various elements, including both organic and inorganic components. The organic parts, which make up approximately 30% of bone mass, consist mainly of collagen fibers, proteoglycans, and other proteins. The inorganic parts, account for the remaining 70%, and are primarily hydroxyapatite crystals (a form of calcium phosphate) and other minerals such as calcium carbonate, magnesium, and fluoride.

Collagen

Collagen is a critical component of bones, providing flexibility and resistance to tensile forces. It forms a network of fibers that create a framework to support minerals and, as a result, the combination of collagen and minerals gives bones both their strength and flexibility. Collagen is also important for skin, nail and hair health, covered in the net chapter, which also details good sources of collagen support.

Proteoglycans and Other Proteins

Proteoglycans and other proteins within bones contribute to their overall structure and integrity. These molecules help regulate the mineralization process and interact with the collagen network to maintain the bone's structural stability.

Hydroxyapatite and Minerals

Hydroxyapatite, a crystalline mineral composed of calcium and phosphate, is responsible for the hardness and rigidity of bones. This mineral, along with other minerals like calcium carbonate and magnesium, contributes to the bone's ability to bear weight and resist compression forces.

Hormones and Bone Health

Hormones play a significant role in bone health throughout life, regulating bone growth, remodeling, and mineralization. The balance of hormones like estrogen, parathyroid hormone (PTH), and calcitonin is essential for maintaining healthy bones - these are covered below.

Parathyroid Hormone (PTH)

Parathyroid hormone (PTH) is secreted by the parathyroid

glands and plays a crucial role in regulating calcium levels in the blood. PTH stimulates the release of calcium from bones, increasing calcium absorption in the intestines, and reducing calcium loss in the kidneys. PTH helps maintain proper calcium levels for various bodily functions, including nerve transmission, muscle contraction, and blood clotting.

Calcitonin

Calcitonin is a hormone produced by the thyroid gland, which acts to lower blood calcium levels. Although its role in overall bone health is less significant than estrogen and PTH, calcitonin helps maintain calcium balance in the body.

What you will notice in all of the above is that calcium keeps cropping up and it's why calcium so important. But calcium alone won't help. You need to combine calcium with vitamin D. Read on!

Estrogen, Progesterone, Osteoclasts and Osteoblasts

Bones are always undergoing a process called "remodelling," which involves the removal of old bone tissue and creation of new tissue. It is so good at this that most of our skeleton will be replaced every 10 years.

This process is carried out by two types of cells: osteoclasts and osteoblasts - osteoclasts are responsible for breaking down old or damaged bone tissue, while osteoblasts are responsible for building new bone tissue.

Estrogen is known to inhibit the activity of osteoclasts, the cells that break down bone tissue. This hormone essentially reduces bone loss by slowing down the rate at which osteoclasts break down bone.

Osteoclasts release enzymes and acids that dissolve the mineral matrix of the bone which then digest the remaining debris (foreign substances, cellular debris, and microorganisms). This process, often overlooked, plays a vital role in the immune systems protection of our body against infections.

It also helps to maintain calcium levels in the body (by helping calcium absorption in the intestines and by reducing calcium loss in the kidneys).

When estrogen levels drop during menopause, this protective effect is reduced, leading to an increase in bone loss.

Meanwhile, progesterone encourages the activity of osteoblasts, the cells that build new bone. It stimulates these cells to produce more bone tissue, normally to help offset the bone loss caused by increased osteoclast activity. They produce and secrete type 1 collagen as well as other proteins that form the organic mix of our bones and release enzymes that eventually result in new bone tissue. They are stimulated by hormones such as calcitonin as well as by mechanical stresses such as weight-bearing exercise.

As progesterone levels decline, the bone building activity slows and as estrogen declines, it is not preventing bone breakdown effectively.

It means that the rate of bone breakdown outpaces bone formation along with a reduction in the release of calcium and collagen.

Meanwhile, we also need Vitamin D to help our body absorb calcium and to help strengthen our bones.

When our skin is exposed to sunlight, a type of cholesterol in our skin cells is converted into vitamin D3. This form of vitamin D then undergoes further processing in the liver and kidneys to become the active form of vitamin D that the body can use.

It's worth noting that the amount of vitamin D that the body can produce through sunlight exposure depends on a number of factors, including time of day, season, latitude, skin tone, and the use of sunscreen.

In some cases, even without menopause, people may not be

able to get enough vitamin D through sunlight alone and may need to supplement their diet with vitamin D-rich foods or take vitamin D supplements. Be careful about taking too much Vitamin D. Too much can cause health issues such as hypercalcemia (abnormally high level of calcium in the blood), nausea, vomiting, and kidney stones.

This is why Calcium, Vitamin D and Collagen are all a part of managing the effects bone health as a result of the menopause.

In essence, estrogen lowers our bone building and so we need calcium and collagen to help support our bone building function, and we need Vitamin D to help our bodies take in the much needed Calcium. This is why, before, during and after menopause your doctor may prescribe Vitamin D, Calcium or Collagen supplements as well as encouraging a calcium rich diet.

And if you are still wondering about phosphorous, estrogen helps to maintain healthy levels of both calcium and phosphorus in the bones and when estrogen levels decline, the body may start breaking down bone tissue to release more calcium and phosphorus into the bloodstream because it's needed elsewhere.

This really matters because approximately 85% of phosphorus in the body is found in bones. It has an important role - it is essential for energy production, pH regulation, and the formation of cell membranes. Progesterone also plays a role in maintaining phosphorus levels. It does this by helping the reabsorption of phosphorus in the kidneys, which helps to maintain the overall balance of phosphorus in the body.

Phosphorus is a mineral that can be found in many foods, including dairy products, meat, fish, and whole grains. It is absorbed from the diet and then processed by the kidneys. Excess phosphorus is excreted in the urine, while any phosphorus that is needed for bone health is deposited in the bones.

Like most things, too much phosphorus in the diet can be

harmful, contributing to kidney disease, cardiovascular disease, and other health problems.

And last but not least, testosterone. This helps to build and maintain bone density and muscle mass and it too plays a crucial role in maintaining bone density in both men and women, as it is converted into estrogen. When testosterone levels drop this too can contribute to bone loss and other complications.

A combination of all of the above can result in the osteoporosis in later life - as the essential hormones and vitamins are lost from our body and we start to break down our bones faster than we can rebuild them.

Other than estrogen, the key things to remember are calcium, vitamin D, collagen and phosphorus. Your body won't absorb that calcium without enough vitamin D. This is because Vitamin D is a fat-soluble vitamin that helps the body absorb calcium from the diet.

Soy, mentioned above, is one of the few plant-based sources of complete protein which is rich in isoflavones, a type of phytoestrogen. These are plant-derived compounds with estrogen-like activity that can (weakly) bind to estrogen receptors in the body. It means it can potentially help some of the symptoms of estrogen decline including helping with hot flashes, as well as potentially reducing the risk of heart disease, joint pain and osteoporosis.

Calcification (Joint Pain)

Calcification is caused by the build-up of calcium salt deposits outside of the bone structure (calcification) rather than the calcium we need inside our bones and it can be very painful and debilitating.

This process can take place in soft tissues such as blood vessels, heart valves, and tendons, or in areas that have previously experienced inflammation or injury. Calcification can also occur within organs like the kidneys, and in this case it can result in kidney stones. It can lead to a range of complications, such as impaired organ function, joint stiffness, and pain.

There are a few causes of calcification and it also effects your blood vessels and heart (cardiovascular calcification) and you will often get mixed advice on whether to avoid calcium or whether to increase your intake.

'Natural' sources of calcium that you find in fruits and vegetables usually provides the 'right' type of calcium but in its additive form it can calcify soft tissue and arteries instead of bone. Calcium supplements can be beneficial for people who have difficulty getting enough calcium through their diet, but it is essential to choose the right type of calcium supplement.

As you might be able to guess, calcification can often start with low estrogen which ends up causing an imbalance between bone breakdown and re-growth - calcification can be one of the side effects.

Sunlight (which helps produce vitamin D3) can even help, but not vitamin D2, which is less effective in raising blood levels of vitamin D. Phosphorus and Collagen both a part of this process too. In some cases reducing over-use of some types of calcium "might" help, exercise can help (weight bearing), Vitamin D3 might help (it helps release proteins/hormones that are needed), as might Vitamin K (which contains MGP protein) as well as considering a diet of anti-inflammatory foods, or, at least, avoiding ones that trigger inflammation.

Be mindful that too much salt can cause high blood pressure (Borex for example) and too much vitamin D, or the wrong kind, might have other effects.

Vitamin K has been proven to help with vascular calcification and castor oil packs have been proven to help reduce pain. Maybe start with finding out if there is a Vitamin K deficiency and ease the pain with the castor oil packs.

General Strategies for Healthy Bones

There are several strategies that you can apply to promote strong and healthy bones as you age. These include:

1. Smoking and excessive alcohol consumption can both contribute to bone loss and osteoporosis. If you smoke, quitting can help promote bone health. Limit alcohol consumption to no more than one drink per day.
2. Weight-bearing exercise refers to any activity that requires your bones to support your body weight, such as walking, jogging, dancing, or weight lifting. When you engage in weight-bearing exercise, your bones experience a mild stress that stimulates the production of new bone tissue, which can help to strengthen and preserve bone mass. Aim for at least 30 minutes of weight-bearing exercise per day. If you are already suffering from joint pain then swimming and yoga are best and because some exercises like weightlifting or running can put a significant amount of stress on sensitive joints like the knees and shoulders they should be done in moderation.
3. Consume a diet that is rich in calcium and vitamin D. Calcium is a mineral that is essential for building and maintaining strong bones, while vitamin D helps your body to absorb calcium. Good dietary sources of calcium include dairy products, leafy green vegetables, and calcium-fortified foods such as orange juice and cereal. Vitamin D is found in fatty fish, egg yolks, and fortified foods, as well as in your skin when it is exposed to sunlight. Women over 50 should aim for 1,200 mg of calcium and 800-1,000 IU of vitamin D per day.

4. Exercise really can help with bone health. Bones grow stronger with exposure to loads and forces

5. Anti-inflammaory foods can help if you are experiencing joint pain. These include fruit and vegetables, whole grains, omega-3 fatty acids, oily fish, nuts and seeds and even dark chocolate!

Bone health exercises

Weight bearing

These types of exercise mean that you are using your feet and legs to support your weight. This can include walking, running or jogging, dancing, aerobics, tennis, badminton

Strength

In this case you are exercising your muscles so that they 'pull' on your bones. These an include press ups, weight training (with or without resistance bands), and pilates. Only do these in moderation if you are already suffering from joint pain.

In addition to exercise and nutrition, there are also several medical treatments available for osteoporosis and joint pain.

Hormone replacement therapy (HRT) can, of course, be effective for preventing bone loss and reducing the risk of bone fracture in postmenopausal women.

Other medications, such as bisphosphonates and denosumab, can also help to slow down bone loss and reduce fracture risk.

If you are worried then you can get regular bone density scans, such as DEXA scans, which can help detect bone loss and osteoporosis early, when treatment is most effective.

Have a blood test to establish which vitamins you are deficient in. Once you know this, you can start by focusing there.

In terms of herbal remedies then the following have some evidence of helping with symptoms:

Mentioned already, Soy is rich in isoflavones, a type of phytoestrogen, which is believed to have estrogen-like effects. Some studies have found that soy isoflavones may slightly increase bone mineral density in postmenopausal women and could potentially slow bone loss. The effect appears to be modest and more research is needed (Taku et al., 2010).

Red Clover, like Soy, it is rich in isoflavones. A 2004 study published in the American Journal of Clinical Nutrition found that daily supplements of red clover isoflavones may slow bone loss and even boost bone mineral density in pre- and peri-menopausal women. More research is still needed to confirm these effects (Atkinson et al., 2004) but it is encouraging.

Black Cohosh is a herb traditionally used to alleviate menopausal symptoms, and research suggests it might help slow bone loss. Be careful with this herb if you have any kidney problems.

Horsetail has been used traditionally as a herbal remedy for osteoporosis, mainly because it's rich in silicon, a mineral needed for bone health. The evidence supporting its effectiveness is still limited (Rondanelli et al., 2019).

Osteoporosis and arthritis

Osteoporosis and arthritis are both conditions that can affect the bones and joints, but they are distinct in their causes, effects, and treatment.

Osteoporosis, often called 'Brittle Bones', is characterised by decreased bone density and strength, and it leads to fragile bones that are more prone to fractures. It is often 'silent' until a bone fracture occurs and the bone doesn't only fracture but can break in multiple places, even with a small fall. As we know it's caused by an imbalance between new bone formation and old bone resorption caused by the declining levels of estrogen. The effect of this can takes years to reveal themselves.

Arthritis, on the other hand, is a general term for conditions that cause joint pain and inflammation and it includes many different types of arthritis, including osteoarthritis and rheumatoid arthritis.

While the relationship with estrogen is less clear-cut than with osteoporosis, it's known that women are more likely to develop rheumatoid arthritis than men. Some research suggests that the drop in estrogen during menopause could potentially contribute to the onset or progression of rheumatoid arthritis.

Arthritis is a degenerative joint disease where the cartilage that cushions the ends of bones within joints gradually wears away. This can lead to pain, stiffness, and loss of joint movement. It's usually a result of aging, but it can also be caused by joint injury or obesity. It's more common in women, particularly after age 50. I wonder why? This is the average age of menopause which suggests - at the very least - that hormonal changes may have a role.

In terms of their relationship, osteoporosis and arthritis can sometimes coexist, especially as they are both more common with advancing age. Additionally, some treatments for arthritis, such as corticosteroids, can increase the risk of osteoporosis. Also, reduced mobility due to arthritis can lead to decreased bone density and muscle mass, which can further exacerbate osteoporosis.

It's also worth noting that osteoarthritis, which is characterised by the wearing down of joint cartilage, can sometimes be associated with increased bone density near the joints, which is the opposite of osteoporosis.

If you are suffering from joint pain it could be the result of arthritis and also the effects of lower hormones as a result of menopause i.e. the conditions can co-exist. Or it could be one or the other that is causing the pain. But, taking a biological supplement in some form (either as HRT if that is your choice, or an alternative) can often help with the pain and discomfort. Importantly, for the longer term impact, many doctors believe that managing hormone levels during peri-menopause and early menopause can make a significant difference to your long terms risk of osteoporosis and harsher arthritis effects and pain. This is one of the reason many women opt to start HRT sooner rather than later. It has been proven to help with this condition and can play a major role in your ability to live a full like in later years.

Herbal Remedies

Arthritis and Joint Pain

Turmeric contains a compound called curcumin, which has anti-inflammatory and antioxidant properties that may help to reduce joint pain and inflammation. Turmeric can be consumed as a spice in food or taken as a supplement. According to the Arthritis Foundation it is safer to choose curcumin extract because whole turmeric can be contaminated with lead. After checking with your doctor, 500 mg capsules twice daily. Also check the standardised amount of curcumin when looking for a supplement, and aim to select brands that use phospholipids (Meriva, BCM-95), antioxidants (CircuWin) or nanoparticles (Theracurmin) for better absorption.

Ginger is another spice that has anti-inflammatory properties and may help to reduce joint pain and stiffness. It can be consumed as a tea, added to food, or taken as a supplement. Studies have confirmed that a daily dose of 500 to 1,000 mg of ginger extract can modestly reduce pain and disability in hip and knee OA.

Willow bark contains a compound called salicin, which is similar to aspirin and has anti-inflammatory and pain-relieving properties. It can be taken as a supplement or brewed into a tea. Some herbal products have been used topically for OA. A 2013 study found that Arnica and Comfrey extract gel might be helpful, and that Capsicum extract gel probably isn't. The evidence on other products was insufficient to allow any firm conclusions to be reached.

Acupuncture may help relieve osteoarthritis pain and there is some evidence (although small) that suggests that massage therapy may be helpful.

Moringa leaves are often used to combat inflammation and osteoarthritis.

Rheumatoid arthritis

Rheumatoid arthritis (RA) is an autoimmune disease and is caused by the immune system attacking healthy cells in our body which leads to inflammation and damage in the joints. In people with RA, immune cells mistakenly target the synovium, the thin membrane that lines the joints, causing inflammation and swelling that can eventually result in joint damage.

While not exclusively the result of lowering estrogen - it can also be genetic for example - it is more common in women and it is thought that and changes in estrogen levels during menopause play a role in this.

While Arthritis and Rheumatoid arthritis can cause joint pain and inflammation, there are some key differences between arthritis and rheumatoid arthritis:

- Arthritis can be caused by a variety of factors, including wear and tear, injury, infection, and autoimmune disorders. Rheumatoid arthritis is specifically caused by an autoimmune response.
- While both types of arthritis can cause joint pain, stiffness, and swelling, rheumatoid arthritis tends to

affect multiple joints at once, and can also cause fatigue, fever, and weight loss.

- Arthritis can progress slowly over time, while rheumatoid arthritis can progress more rapidly, causing more severe joint damage and disability.
- Treatment for arthritis depends on the underlying cause, but may include pain relief medications, physical therapy, and lifestyle changes. Treatment for rheumatoid arthritis typically involves medications that suppress the immune system to reduce inflammation and slow the progression of the disease.

Nobody knows exactly what causes this autoimmune disease, but if rheumatoid arthritis is not treated, it can lead to the complete destruction of your joints. There is no cure for rheumatoid arthritis, there are rarely are cures for autoimmune diseases, but there are ways to treat the inflammation and pain.

Here are six herbs that you can try:

- **Cinnamon** – Studies have shown that cinnamon powder, when consumed in capsules, can help to reduce inflammation. You can also incorporate cinnamon into your cooking if you prefer.
- **Garlic** – Not only can garlic reduce inflammation, but it may also be able to protect the cartilage around your joints. You can use garlic capsules, but it may be just as effective (and a lot more enjoyable) to add fresh garlic to your meals.
- **Willow Bark** – A 2013 study found that willow bark was highly effective in the treatment of rheumatoid arthritis. It contains salicin, which is similar to aspirin, and has anti-inflammatory properties which can help reduce the symptoms of autoimmune disorders like rheumatoid arthritis. It was also found to be effective

for several other musculoskeletal disorders. A tincture may work, but tablets of powdered willow bark tend to be most effective. Talk to your doctor before using them.

- **Green Tea** – Another powerful anti-inflammatory, green tea has many uses and is a great drink. You can, of course, take green tea supplements, but a cup of green tea is always a nice way to enjoy this wonderful herb.

- **Ginger** – The final anti-inflammatory remedy on this list, ginger is a well-known at being effective in reducing inflammation and it can help reduce pain and swelling in the joints caused by the injury. It is best to add ginger into your diet, but you can also consume it in capsule form if you prefer.

- **Cat's Claw** - The Journal of Rheumatology published a study of Cat's Claw for the treatment of RA. Researchers found that in 40 people with RA, the supplement reduced joint swelling and pain by more than 50 percent compared to placebo. You can take as capsules, tablets, and tea. 250 mg to 350 mg capsule daily for immune support. Use products that contain uncaria tomentosa and make sure it is free of tetracyclic oxindole alkaloids (TOAs).

These same herbs can be used for the other forms of arthritis. Acupuncture has been used in Traditional Chinese Medicine for a very long time. Western medicine is still highly skeptical about its abilities, but many people with rheumatoid arthritis swear by it as a form of short-term pain relief.

As sleep can be such an effective way of reducing the symptoms of rheumatoid arthritis, it may be a good idea to look at herbal remedies to improve your sleep. **Lavender** essential oil is a good start; **Valerian** root supplements can also help. Take a look at the chapter on sleep for more strategies that can help with insomnia.

Psoriatic arthritis

Psoriatic arthritis is a type of arthritis that is associated with psoriasis, a skin condition that often reveals itself as red, scaly patches on the skin.

The exact cause of psoriatic arthritis is not known, but it is also believed to be an autoimmune disorder. The symptoms of psoriatic arthritis include joint pain, stiffness, and swelling, as well as skin lesions.

Again, a herbal remedy won't cure this condition, but there are a few that might be helpful and two of these are **Aloe vera** is a plant that has anti-inflammatory and analgesic properties and may help to reduce joint pain and inflammation. It can be applied topically as a gel or taken as a supplement.

The ever useful **Turmeric**, as mentioned earlier, also has anti-inflammatory and antioxidant properties and may be helpful for reducing joint pain and inflammation in psoriatic arthritis.

Overall, if you can't or don't want to take either HRT or other medications for bone health, then you want to consider herbs or supplements that contain Omega-3, glucosamine (and Chondroitin), Manganese (which supports Collagen formation in the cartilage, tendons and ligaments), along with the vitamins mentioned earlier - ideally with knowledge of any weakness of a particular vitamin in your blood.

TEN

GSM: Vaginal Health and The Libido, Pelvis and Urinary Tract

P erhaps one of the worst names ever given to a menopause symptom is 'Vaginal atrophy'. A horrible name but it's also a horrible problem. It actually refers to the group of conditions now called Genitourinary syndrome of menopause (GSM) and is the new term for vulvovaginal atrophy (VVA). It covers conditions effecting the vagina, vulva, pelvic floor tissues, urinary tract, and sexual dysfunction and loss of libido. I go onto to talk about the pelvic and urinary impact in the next chapter, but here I am going to focus on the vagina and your libido.

It sounds like a very complicated condition but the cause is actually very simple - it's the result of low estrogen levels. This causes a myriad of problems that centre around the thinning of the vaginal and urinary tissues causing, for example, the vagina to become less elastic and, at the same time, lowering mucous production. It is this lack of lubrication which causes vaginal dryness, soreness, itching, burning and painful sex. And it's extremely uncomfortable and can be debilitating. I have heard it described as like having sandpaper between your legs and some women have difficulty walking at all.

This is one of the least discussed affects of the loss of our hormones as we travel through midlife, yet it is arguably far-and-away, the symptom that impacts many, many (if not most) women and it can have have the biggest long-term debilitating impact on our life. We need to start talking about it.

In Australia, the Royal Australian College of General Practitioners reports that 50% of women have an "adverse impact on quality of life, social activity and sexual relationships" because of GSM. In the UK Dr Louise Newson says as many as 80% of women suffer from dry vulvas (and only 8% seek help). It really is a case of suffering in silence. A Women's Health Initiative Study found that 60% of participants had physical evidence of vaginal atrophy, but only 10% declared they had symptoms. Worse, it was estimated that only 7% of women were treated.

It doesn't help that, for example, a recent report said that as few as 20% of OB-GYN's 's in the US have been trained in menopause symptoms. And the US is not alone. Many women discover that if they see a doctor for vaginal pain they will be prescribed antibiotics for a urinary tract infection - I know at least 3 personally - and this is the case the more-or-less across the world.

But, it isn't only lack of knowledge of the treatment available- its embarrassment of both the patient and the doctor. Women often wait for their healthcare professional to ask the 'right' questions while the healthcare professionals are embarrassed or scared to ask the difficult questions particularly about sex. This can be harder for younger male doctors who don't like asking a 50 or 60 something woman about their vagina and especially about sex. Many others dismiss the symptoms as part of normal ageing.

This is the easiest of all problems to solve. Talk.

And the solution is easy. The best is simply estrogen replacement - specifically topical vaginal estrogen or pessaries which I go on to discuss later in this chapter. This solution can be used by anyone even those who have breast cancer because the dose is so small.

The great news is, if you live in the UK, as of April 2023, you can now get an over-the-counter HRT called Gina for vaginal dryness and pain. You will still need to talk to a qualified pharmacist because its not off-the-shelf but you no longer need a prescription. It's called Gina 10 microgram vaginal tablets and it contains estradiol - it won't work on any other symptoms - it is purely for vaginal dryness.

Vaginal Dryness

Vulval burning, dryness, irritation or itching are some of the vulval symptoms that make up the term GSM and specifically vaginal dryness. As well as making day-to-life difficult or unbearable also makes sex painful, so much so, that it is avoided altogether.

One reason for this is something medically described as "entry dyspareunia with fissuring". It means pain during sexual intercourse, specifically when penetration is attempted. Fissuring, or small tears or cracks in the skin, can happen as a result of the skin in this area becoming thinner and drier as a result of lower oestrogen, and this one of the reasons that you can experience pain during sex.

And don't think for a second that vaginal dryness is a problem limited to peri menopause or the early stages of menopause - nor indeed think that estrogen replacement can't help you at any age.

Again in Australia, the Melbourne Women's Midlife Study, found that it actually increased with age with 4% experiencing vaginal dryness in early perimenopause, "rising to 25% at one year postmenopause and 47% three years after the menopause. And the symptoms range from mild, moderate to debilitating."

Other studies have found that 50% of women aged 50–60

years report symptoms, increasing to 72% in women aged older than 70 years, yet only 4% associated their symptoms with loss of oestrogen at menopause. (The Royal Australian College of General Practitioners).

Estrogen is the food of the vulva - it keeps the blood flowing, helps collagen and elastin production. That latter two help give tissue its structure and elasticity, keeping things elastic but firm - while supporting the production of the vaginal fluids. Testosterone also plays a role here too.

The reduction in the number of blood vessels happens because oestrogen influences blood vessel growth and health. Fewer blood vessels can lead to less blood flow to the tissue, which can contribute to a thinning of the tissue surface (the epithelium) and decrease its elasticity, which means it becomes less able to return to its original shape after being stretched or contracted.

Testosterone and progesterone also plays a role here too - not such a big role, but a role none-the-less. But progesterone won't be of help with vaginal dryness.

Estrogen receptors are present in the vagina, the vulva, urethra and bladder. Meanwhile, testosterone receptors are concentrated mainly in the vulval tissues and progesterone receptors are found in the vagina and at the 'vulvovaginal epithelial junction'. The term "vulvovaginal epithelial junction" may sound a bit like a science textbook, but it's really not as complicated as it sounds.

The 'vulvo-' part refers to the vulva, which is the external part of a woman's genital area. This includes the lips around the vagina (labia), the clitoris, and the openings of the vagina and urethra.

The '-vaginal' part, as you might guess, refers to the vagina, the internal passage leading from the vulva up to the uterus or womb.

'Epithelial' refers to the type of cells that make up the outer and inner linings of our body's cavities and surfaces – it's like the body's wallpaper. The epithelial cells in this case are those lining the vulva and vagina.

The 'junction' is just where two things meet or join. So, the "vulvovaginal epithelial junction" is simply the place where the lining of the vulva meets the lining of the vagina. It's a sort of borderland where the outside and inside meet, a bridge between the external and internal parts of a woman's intimate area.

Changes in vaginal epithelial cells describes how the cells that line the vagina also change with menopause. Without covering all the science, it can cause further thinning and changes in the tissue as estrogen reduces.

Vaginal dryness causes a host of problem and can contribute to prolapse, fused labia and urinary infections. One other problem that was pointed out more than once by women as that this condition also made the Cervical Smear Test painful. It's well worth finding a remedy that works for you.

Urinary Health and Your Bladder

Urinary problems can make it pain its painful to go to the loo, but also it can make you want to find the ladies as fast as possible. It can result in leaks

Urinary discomfort can often persist into your sixties, sometimes even starting then, and can frequently be mistaken for cystitis. Your vagina, like your gut, has a 'healthy microbiome,' or beneficial bacteria.

This means that Urinary Tract Infections (UTIs) can make an appearance. Estrogen helps maintain a healthy balance of good bacteria in the urethra, which can help prevent harmful bacteria from causing infections. As estrogen levels drop, this balance can be disrupted, making it easier for harmful bacteria to take hold and cause an infection. Symptoms of a UTI can include a strong urge to urinate, a burning sensation during urination, cloudy or strong-smelling urine, and pelvic pain. But, take note, antibiotics often won't help. The problem is caused by the lack of estrogen.

Estrogen supports this microbiome, and as its levels decline, we lose its protective function as well as its role in mucus production. Like our gut, probiotics like Kefir can help here, but they won't solve the root of the problem.

In addition to this, there is the thinning of the urinary tract wall and weakening of our muscles as we outline above. This can be when physical activity like coughing, sneezing, or exercising causes urine to leak, where a sudden, intense urge to urinate is followed by an involuntary loss of urine. The decrease in estrogen weakens the urinary sphincter, the muscle that controls the release of urine from the bladder, making it harder to control urination.

Pelvis and Prolapse

And so we now reach the pelvis and the problem of prolapse. This, along with a fused labia, can all start with vaginal dryness along with the reduction in estrogen.

It happens when the muscles and tissues supporting the pelvic organs (the uterus, bladder, and rectum) become weak or loose, and this weakening can cause one or more of the pelvic organs to drop or press into or out of the vagina. Once again, it's the decrease in estrogen which weakens these muscles and tissues, making it more likely for you to experience pelvic organ prolapse.

Along with estrogen replacement, exercises can really help here, and the earlier you start support your pelvic muscles the better. If you aren't suffering from vaginal dryness or a weak bladder then yoga can be great for the pelvic area. Many of you will have done pelvic exercises after giving birth, dig them out and do them again.

Pelvic Floor Exercises

Pelvic floor exercises are specifically targeted exercises to strengthen the muscles supporting the bladder, uterus, and bowels. These exercises, commonly known as Kegels, can improve bladder control and reduce symptoms of urinary incontinence.

If you are also suffering with constipation (yet another symptom), cut back on caffeine and drink more water. Caffeine can help with constipation but in this case, it's better to try other solutions.

Regular exercise can help reduce pelvic pain by improving blood circulation, releasing endorphins (natural pain-relieving hormones), and promoting overall muscle strength and flexibility.

Don't forget to avoid exercise that puts stress on the pelvic floor, for example, aerobics, jogging - any high impact activity - and take up exercises that squeeze and lift.

The Libido

Before I discuss the importance of estrogen or other possible remedies we need to discuss the libido. You can already see that everything is linked - and I am pretty sure you knew that before you read this book - so let's take a look at what's going on with our libido.

It's pretty clear that the problems with vaginal dryness and all the other associated problems are not going to help with any libido problems. But your libido also has another hormone that is dampening its enthusiasm. And that is the hormone often thought to be male-only, testosterone.

I'm going to get this one over with right away. Orgasms. Believe it or not but orgasms can really help - accompanied or unaccompanied. Orgasms release dopamine and oxytocin which are great for the immune system and mental health, balancing the stress hormone cortisol, as well as boosting blood flow to the vagina. It get's better. You need to start early! The more you can do during peri menopause or earlier, the better.

You will help keep the blood flowing to your vulva as your estrogen is declining - giving it a helping hand, so-to-speak. On top of that it will boost your happy hormone levels (dopamine and oxytocin as well as cortisol) which can help your mental health along with sleep (it can even help with migraines).

Chronic stress, the insidious saboteur, ties into hormonal imbalances, disrupting thyroid function and dwindling reserves of sex hormones like estrogen and testosterone. Current research suggests testosterone can offer a modest boost to sexual desire, pleasure, arousal, and orgasm frequency.

If non-medical solutions are ineffective, remember: testosterone should be administered in doses that elevate levels to those typical in premenopausal women. At these doses, the primary side effects are typically limited to mild acne and increased facial hair.

Sadly, as of 2021, the FDA in the U.S. hadn't given testosterone its blessing for managing low libido in women. In fact, there wasn't an FDA-approved product on the market catering to women with dwindling libido.

If you can't get hold of testosterone or estrogen, or you don't want to, then certain herbs, such as maca and ginseng, are touted for their libido-boosting properties.

And let's not neglect the potential of professional help. Therapists and counsellors skilled in sexual health issues can provide valuable insights and techniques to help restore your libido. You might also consider joining a support group of women going through similar experiences - sometimes, simply knowing that you're not alone can provide immense relief.

Finally, don't underestimate the power of open communication and emotional intimacy. If libido loss is causing concern, discussing these feelings with your partner can be immensely therapeutic. Also, remember that physical intimacy isn't just about sex. Touching, cuddling, and other forms of contact can be just as satisfying and affirming.

The Solutions To Your Problems

Now that I have explained as much as you probably want to know, it's time to find out what can help.

Needless to say, many of the problems begin with the whole area of vaginal dryness, a deflated vulva, limited lubrication, thinning skin, all resulting in pain, discomfort, and feelings of failure. None of these can be under-estimated in terms of the impact it can have on our life, our mental health and our overall joie de vivre.

Estrogen is a trusty ally in the fight against dryness. Both pills and patches of the hormone can help alleviate dryness, mitigate sexual discomfort, and bolster overall sexual function. Topical solutions applied straight to the problem area can be the most and, indeed, many menopause specialists tip their hats to the direct approach, recommending such topical applications. On the flip side, progesterone doesn't aid in mitigating sexual pain.

Research brings another hero to the fore: vaginal lubricants sans estrogen. Both plant-based and silicone-based lubricants may ease your primary complaints—dryness and discomfort during sex and it's worth considering lubricants to determine if they lessen your discomfort.

Don't disregard the potential role of diet. Foods rich in omega-3 fatty acids, like fish, chia seeds, flaxseeds, and walnuts, can provide natural lubrication, helping your body to maintain healthy moisture levels. And drink lots of water too.

You can also explore phytoestrogens, naturally occurring compounds found in a wide variety of foods. They mimic the function of estrogen to a certain extent, foods rich in these compounds - such as soy products, flaxseeds, and certain fruits and vegetables - can offer some help.

In terms of vaginal dryness and pain that's not associated with sex, estrogen pills and patches can offer relief. Just remember: progesterone won't be of help here.

If dryness persists despite these measures, consider speaking to a healthcare professional. They could prescribe topical treatments that contain hyaluronic acid or vitamin E, both of which are known to soothe and hydrate the vaginal area. One of the best methods of using HRT for vaginal dryness is as a pessary. The estrogen is delivered in tiny amounts directly to your skin which means it is both extremely effective and safe for almost all women.

If you have decided not to use HRT, or can't us HRT, to replace your estrogen and progesterone, then there are a number of other strategies that you can adopt to help with your symptoms. Even if you are taking HRT you might want to incorporate some or all of the following.

Natural remedies

Herbal supplements like black cohosh and evening primrose oil, and making dietary adjustments to include more plant-based foods. Explore natural remedies, such as coconut oil or vitamin E, to moisturize and soothe the vaginal area.

Diet and Nutrition

Incorporate foods rich in phytoestrogens, such as soy products, flaxseeds, and lentils, which can help balance hormone levels. Avoid trigger foods like caffeine, spicy foods, alcohol, spicy foods, artificial sweeteners, and acidic foods like citrus fruits and tomatoes which can all irritate the bladder and worsen symptoms.

Stress Management and Mindfullness

High stress levels can lead to increased muscle tension, hormone imbalances, and heightened sensitivity to pain while stress, anxiety, and poor self-esteem are frequent culprits behind a dwindling sex drive. Incorporating stress management practices such as mindfulness, meditation, yoga, and deep-breathing exercises into your routine or engaging in hobbies that bring you joy and relaxation can be invaluable.

ELEVEN

The Weight Balancing Act

There are so many elements that effect our weight at the time of menopause, as falling estrogen changes the way fat is distributed around out body. From low energy levels, poor sleep, weakening muscles and our heart health. The impact on weight is covered over quite a few chapters but it's worthwhile understanding a bit more about what's going on.

On its own, estrogen plays a significant role in various physiological processes, including metabolism and fat distribution. It influences how the body uses and stores energy, it helps regulate glucose and lipid metabolism, which are crucial for maintaining energy balance in the body. Changes in these metabolic signals, often due to estrogen deficiency, can lead to metabolic syndrome and a higher risk of cardiovascular disease. We also know that the loss of estrogen with menopause shifts fat tissue accumulation away from the lower body towards our central/abdominal areas.

Estrogen receptors, which are proteins that bind to estrogen, are found in various tissues, including fat tissue and they play a key role in metabolic regulation. When estrogen binds to these receptors, it triggers a series of events that influence metabolic processes. It affects where fat is stored in the body and how fat cells, or adipocytes, differentiate and function. It impacts glucose (energy levels) and our lipids - which increase our abdominal fat accumulation.

Post-menopausal women often experience an increase in abdominal fat accumulation, and it is this which is associated with a higher risk of metabolic and cardiovascular diseases.

However, the relationship between estrogen deficiency and obesity is complex and not fully understood.

Then we have something known as 'lipedema'. It affects over 1 in 10 woman (estimates range from 11–19%) and even these estimates are thought to understate the true prevalence of this disease given its frequency of misdiagnosis and late diagnosis according to the study "Current Mechanistic Understandings of Lymphedema and Lipedema"). It strikes during periods of hormonal fluctuation, such as puberty, pregnancy, or menopause and can be triggered by use of hormonal birth control pills.

This condition is commonly known as "pear-shaped" body fat distribution where the lower part is wider than the top because of the deposits of fat beneath the skin typically in the legs and lower body. It's a chronic condition that can be painful and can significantly impact the quality of life and it can often be mistaken for mistaken conditions such as lymphedema (swelling of the lower limbs) and, in most severe cases, general obesity.

We don't really know for sure what the cause is but research indicates that its possibly genetic too and its when to too much fat (adipose tissue) squeezes our small blood vessels. This can cause more protein and fluid to build up in the spaces between cells. Our lymphatic vessels help get rid of extra fluid, but if you have lipedema, these vessels also get squished by the extra fat, making it even harder for the body to remove the extra fluid from the lower limbs (like the legs, hips, thighs and buttocks).

It is distinct from obesity because of this specific fat distribution and, unlike obesity that occurs at any stage of life, lipedema only tends to occur during times of hormonal fluctuation.

Now, I don't have an answer for you here! We really don't know for sure what the root cause is nor a sure-fire way to help (there is no known cure).

It also isn't clear what effect HRT has on lipedema fat during menopause but it is often recommended that you avoid high dose Hormone Replacement Therapy if you are suffering from lipedema. This is not a research-based advice nor medical advice, but I would err on the side of avoiding HRT if I personally had this condition.

It's confusing because, according to an older 2014 survey by Lipoedema UK, (this is the UK spelling) the majority of affected women have already developed lipedema by the time they reach menopause. It found that 4% of the women taking part said their lipedema symptoms first appeared at the time of menopause. This could well be related to hormone based birth control but we just don't know. What is likely is that there is an existing genetic condition that makes the hormonal effects more pronounced.

This isn't a book about lipedema, but it's a great example of how much we need to learn about women's health.

For example, from the Australian research the 3 most effective pain relievers were MLD or LDM - Manual Lymphatic Drainage - a gentle form of skin stretching/massage (45%), compression garments (43%), then some way behind Liposuction (38%). The least effective were Diet (other) at 15% followed by Mediterranean diet (16%) then Weight loss sugary (18%). In terms of helping shape the top 3 were Resection/lift (67%), but this only helped 21% with pain, then liposuction (65%) then compression garments at 41%. Those that were the least effective with shape were supplements, and then a tie between yoga/breathing and medications. Overall covering both shape and pain the most ineffective treatments tried were diet and supplements/medications.

"For years, I have lived with lipoedema, and been told that diet and exercise was the path to better health. Now, science is starting to explain why I could never curb my body's excess fat production through lifestyle controls. I am not obese and have a real medical condition that needs treatment. This research is exactly the kind of breakthrough that people like me have been waiting for. It provides renewed hope for me, that my children may not have to suffer the way I have suffered all my life." **Nola Young, Chair Lipoedema Australia.**

If you have lipedema, then diet and exercise is unlikely to help relieve the pain or solve your shape - as far as we know right now. The best advice here is to find out if someone in your family has had this condition and try compression garments and massage to find out if that helps. Testing is difficult because it involves ruling out other conditions rather than confirming a positive test for lipedema - but it is possible.

However, there is some good news for typical menopausal weight gain. That's the bulge then develops around your middle. Although I still find it hard to recommend HRT for weight gain problems alone.

For typical menopause weight gain, it really is down to diet and lifestyle, reducing inflammation, and supporting your blood vessels and so on. All of this is covered in Part II coming up next.

Chapter Resources

Current Mechanistic Understandings of Lymphedema and Lipedema https://www.mdpi.com/1422-0067/22/21/11720

Estrogen Deficiency and the Origin of Obesity during Menopause https://www.ncbi.nlm.nih.gov/pmc/articles/PMC3964739/

Learning by Listening FIRST LOOK Early findings from the Lipedema Foundation Registry survey https://static1.squarespace.com/static/5775899ac534a5e813c050db/t/6290d2cd923a0156d8fcea1e/1653658317504/LF_First+Look+Registry+Report.pdf

Part II: Approaches to Managing Menopause

TWELVE

Hormonal Testing

H ormonal testing and treatment can be an intimidating topic, but it's important to understand the options available and the impact they can have on your health.

From the previous chapters, it should be self-evident that estrogen and a number of other hormones drive our health and well-being and that finding ways to manage, or at the very least, minimise, the impact of the loss of our hormones can make a significant difference to your life.

In the first section, we'll dive into the different types of hormonal testing and what they measure. It's essential to know which tests are relevant to your hormonal concerns and to have a clear understanding of the results. We'll also discuss when it's appropriate to seek medical treatment for hormonal imbalances.

Each woman has different hormone levels, for example, research has found that younger women going through perimenopause or menopause usually need more estradiol. That's why they often need higher doses of hormone replacement therapy (HRT) compared to older women.

The good news is that there are many options available for

hormonal testing and treatment, both natural and conventional. In this chapter, we'll explore the different types of hormonal testing, how to interpret your results, and the various treatment options available.

Understanding Hormonal Testing

Hormonal testing is an essential part of assessing hormonal imbalances. These tests can help identify the underlying causes of your symptoms and determine the best course of treatment. There are several different types of tests available, including blood tests, saliva tests, and urine tests. Each test measures different hormones and can provide different insights into your hormonal health.

You usually don't need blood tests to figure out if you're in peri menopause or menopause. That's because these tests, which check your hormone levels, can be unreliable. This is particularly true during peri menopause, when your hormone levels can change a lot. Very generally, and fluctuations aside, if you are under 40 then at least two blood tests are recommended and if both show elevated FSH (the estrogen stimulating hormone) then this can indicate that you are peri-menopausal.

But these hormone blood tests can sometimes be helpful for women who are using hormone replacement therapy (HRT). They can help check how well your body is absorbing the hormones from the HRT.

Estradiol levels can be used to see how well your body is absorbing hormone replacement therapy (HRT). These levels aren't very accurate if you're taking estrogen as a pill, because your body changes the estrogen into different forms when it digests the pill. But if you're using HRT on your skin (transdermal HRT), these levels can help to make sure your body is properly absorbing the treatment through your skin. This is especially important if you're still having symptoms.

If you're still having symptoms even though you're taking HRT, it might mean something else is the causes. That's why it's always important to talk to a healthcare professional if you're having symptoms.

Types of Hormonal Testing and What They Measure

Blood tests are one of the most common types of hormonal testing. These tests measure the levels of hormones in your blood and can help identify imbalances in hormone production or regulation.

Common hormones measured in blood tests include thyroid hormones, sex hormones (estrogen, progesterone, testosterone), and cortisol.

Saliva tests are another type of hormonal testing. These tests measure the levels of hormones in your saliva and are typically used to assess sex hormone levels. Saliva tests can provide a more accurate reflection of hormone levels than blood tests because they measure the levels of free, or unbound, hormones that are more biologically active than the bound hormones in your bloodstream.

Urine tests are also used to assess hormonal imbalances. These tests measure the levels of hormones and their metabolites in your urine. Urine tests can provide insight into how your body is metabolising and eliminating hormones, which can be useful in identifying imbalances.

Imaging tests like ultrasounds, MRIs, and CT scans can be used to visualise organs like the thyroid and ovaries and identify any structural abnormalities or growths that may be affecting hormone production.

Interpreting Hormonal Test Results

Interpreting hormonal test results can be complicated, and

it's important to work with a qualified healthcare provider to ensure that you're getting the right treatment for your individual needs. Some factors that can affect hormone levels include age, sex, and overall health.

For example, a 35-year-old woman may have different hormonal needs than a 55-year-old woman. Hormonal testing can provide insight into these individual needs and help identify imbalances that may be contributing to symptoms such as mood swings, hot flashes, or fatigue.

While it's common for women's estrogen levels to decline as they age, there is no one-size-fits-all approach to hormone replacement therapy (HRT). Your healthcare provider will consider your individual needs, symptoms, and health history to determine whether HRT is appropriate for you and what type of HRT may be best.

It's also important to understand that hormone levels can fluctuate throughout the day and throughout the menstrual cycle. Hormonal tests may need to be repeated over time to get an accurate picture of your hormone levels.

When interpreting hormonal test results, it's essential to consider not only the levels of individual hormones but also their ratios.

Another important hormonal test is the cortisol test, which measures levels of the stress hormone cortisol in the blood or saliva. Cortisol levels naturally fluctuate throughout the day and can be affected by factors such as stress, sleep, and exercise. However, consistently high or low levels of cortisol can indicate a problem with the adrenal glands, which produce cortisol.

Interpreting cortisol test results can be challenging because cortisol levels can vary widely depending on the time of day and other factors. Typically, cortisol levels should be highest in the morning and gradually decrease throughout the day. A cortisol test result that shows consistently high cortisol levels can indicate Cushing's syndrome, a condition in which the body produces too much cortisol. On the other hand, consistently low cortisol levels can indicate Addison's disease, a condition in which the adrenal glands do not produce enough cortisol.

Other hormonal tests may measure levels of estrogen, progesterone, testosterone, follicle-stimulating hormone (FSH), luteinising hormone (LH), and more. For example, a high level of FSH and a low level of estrogen can indicate menopause or premature ovarian failure, while a high level of LH and a low level of testosterone can indicate polycystic ovary syndrome (PCOS).

Here are some general guidelines for the normal ranges of the hormones mentioned:

In women, estrogen levels can vary widely throughout the menstrual cycle. In the follicular phase (days 1-14), normal levels will be much lower than they are during the luteal phase (days 15-28).

The normal range of estradiol during menstration is 70 pg/mL (250 pmol/L) and usually not higher than 275 pg/mL (1000 pmol/L).

It's important to note that these ranges are general guidelines and can vary depending on the laboratory and specific testing methods used. Additionally, individual results should always be interpreted in the context of a person's medical history and current symptoms - remember that hormonal testing is just one piece of the puzzle when it comes to diagnosing and treating hormonal imbalances.

They are often caused by disruptions in the delicate balance between hormones, rather than absolute levels of individual hormones.

When to Seek Treatment

If you're experiencing symptoms of hormonal imbalance, it's essential to seek medical treatment. Symptoms such as hot flashes, mood swings, or irregular periods can be indicative of hormonal imbalances that require treatment. If left untreated, hormonal imbalances can lead to more severe symptoms and potentially long-term health consequences.

A reminder of some of the common symptoms:

- Irregular menstrual periods or heavy bleeding
- Hot flashes or night sweats
- Mood swings or depression
- Weight gain or difficulty losing weight
- Low libido or sexual dysfunction
- Fatigue or difficulty sleeping
- Hair loss or thinning
- Dry skin or acne

THIRTEEN

HRT and body-identical hormones

B y now you will know how important estrogen and the other hormones, progesterone (and to a lesser degree testosterone) are to almost all of the conditions women experience during and after menopause.

HRT, which stands for Hormone Replacement Therapy, represents the most potent yet misunderstood form of treatment for menopausal symptoms and long-term health.

Taking estrogen to replace some of what is no longer made by the body can offer relief from some symptoms during peri menopause.

Once again take note, women with a uterus need to take a progesterone with the estrogen because estrogen makes the uterine lining grow. Adding progesterone stops this growth and prevents the estrogen from causing uterine cancer.

HRT not only improves quality of life but, the transdermal estrogen in HRT can lead to a longer life reducing the risk of diseases like heart disease, osteoporosis, stroke, colon cancer and Type II diabetes. The longer-term benefits are one of the main reasons I use plant-based body-identical HRT and that's before I mention the support it has in protecting against joint pain and arthritis. It is very hard to understand why the medical profession still seems to be waking up to these longer term benefits.

One of the reasons could, of course, be that plant-based medicine cannot be patented. If you are familiar with herbal medicine then this will not be knew to you. Simply, there is no profit in plant-based remedies.

Navigating the world of hormone replacement therapy (HRT) can feel like a daunting expedition into uncharted territory. You see, one size doesn't fit all when it comes to HRT. The dosage and type of hormones should be tailored to fit your unique circumstances. As in, do you still have your uterus, or was it removed? This factors into whether you'll need progesterone alongside estrogen. Are you prone to certain health risks, such as blood clots or heart disease? This will influence the type of estrogen you'll be recommended. Are you just entering menopause, or have you been postmenopausal for a while? Again, this impacts the treatment strategy.

One common misconception around HRT is the increased risk of breast cancer. However, the key point to grasp is that not all HRT is created equal. Specifically, the form of progesterone used in the treatment is of paramount importance.

There are two main types of progesterone used in HRT. First, the chemically-synthesized version called Progestin, which isn't identical to the natural hormone your body produces, and is associated with an increased risk of breast cancer. And then there's the natural or micronised progesterone, identical to the hormone your body naturally produces, sourced from yams and known as body-identical. This form of progesterone has fewer side effects and has been proven to be safer than its synthetic counterpart.

Does HRT cause cancer?

The controversy surrounding this question originated from a study by The Women's Health Initiative (WHI), which I will discuss shortly. But before that, it is crucial to understand the concepts of progesterone and progestin.

Progesterone exists in two different forms within HRT—natural and chemical. The chemical form, known as Progestin or Progestorgin, is synthesized from testosterone (and occasionally progesterone), but its chemical structure differs from that of our bodies. It is commonly used in contraceptive pills and older forms of HRT, which have been associated with a slight increase in breast cancer risk.

On the other hand, natural or micronized progesterone, which is structurally identical to the body's progesterone, is derived from Yam and is referred to as "body-identical" prog-esterone.

While both forms have a similar effect on the uterine lining, they exhibit nearly opposite effects on other parts of the body, including the breasts and the brain, according to Dr. Lara Briden, the author of the Hormone Repair Manual. This explains why progesterone may be a safer alternative to prog-estin, with potentially more positive effects on mood, hair, skin, and other aspects. Consequently, if you opt for HRT, it is advis-able to choose one that uses progesterone.

This is just one of the reasons why researchers consider the original Women's Health Initiative to be incomplete. The study, initiated in the early 1990s, consisted of two randomized clinical trials investigating the effects of HRT on postmenopausal women.

The focus of the study was on estrogen-alone therapy and combined estrogen-progestin therapy—the older, synthesized form of HRT. The estrogen-progestin trial was prematurely halted in 2002, three years ahead of schedule, due to an increased risk of breast cancer, heart disease, stroke, and blood clots in the HRT group compared to the placebo group. Similarly, the estrogen-alone trial was halted in 2004 due to an increased risk of stroke and no significant impact on heart disease.

Understandably, the WHI study's results caused a significant decline in HRT prescriptions, as many women and healthcare providers became concerned about the associated risks.

However, the study has since been widely discredited. One of the key issues was the age of the participants—many of them were well beyond the age of natural menopause, with an average age of 63 at the start of the trial, approximately 10 to 12 years after the usual onset of menopause. Additionally, some participants had pre-existing heart disease or were at risk of heart disease when they enrolled. The study used a specific type of HRT, namely conjugated equine estrogen (derived from the urine of pregnant horses) and medroxyprogesterone acetate (still used in oral HRT today), These factors limit the study's applicability to all forms of hormone therapy and also employed a one-size-fits-all dosage instead of individualized doses based on each woman's specific needs. It is important to note that the study was observational in nature, meaning it could establish correlations but not causation. While the WHI study highlighted associations between HRT usage and certain health outcomes, it could not definitively prove that HRT caused those outcomes due to the limitations related to participant age and pre-existing conditions.

In response to the WHI study, the Kronos Early Estrogen Prevention Study (KEEPS) was launched. This study included younger women closer to the onset of menopause and used body-identical progesterone. The results? No significant increase in adverse cardiovascular or cognitive events, or breast cancers among the HRT group compared to the placebo group.

KEEPS recruited more than 700 women at low cardiovascular risk who were within three years of their last menstrual period to investigate the cardiovascular, cognitive, and mood effects of two forms of MHT (menopausal hormone therapy)— conjugated estrogen and estradiol — both with oral progesterone.

"During the study, there were no major adverse cardiovascular or cognitive events, or differences in incidence of breast cancers among MHT and placebo groups," said Kejal Kantarci, M.D., a principal investigator in the Department of Radiology at the Mayo Clinic College of Medicine and Science. "This information should provide reassurance to women with low cardiovascular risk who are considering use of hormone treatment to reduce menopausal symptoms."

According to the study "Both forms of MHT reduced the severity of menopausal symptoms, including hot flashes, night sweats, and poor sleep. In addition, the estrogen treatment showed a positive effect on mood, while the estradiol treatment improved sexual function. Both treatments also helped to maintain bone density and decrease insulin resistance."

Unsurprisingly these studies have shown that factors such as age, timing of HRT initiation, and the specific formulation of HRT can influence the overall risk-benefit profile, as well as any underlying medical conditions.

In light of such findings, the "timing hypothesis" has gained traction, suggesting that starting HRT closer to the onset of menopause might actually be beneficial. A recent study published in the JAMA Neurology journal in March 2023 supports this notion, suggesting that starting HRT five or more years after menopause could increase the risk of dementia in women who have experienced early menopause.

"HT (hormone therapy) is the most reliable way to ameliorate severe menopause symptoms, but over the last few decades, there has been a lack of clarity on how HT affects the brain," study corresponding author Rachel Buckley said.

"Hormone therapy can have negative effects on cognition,

but only if initiated several years after age at menopause. These observational findings support clinical guidelines that state hormone therapy should be administered close to menopause onset, but not several years after," study first author Gillian Coughlan said.

This underlines that your choice, and timing, of HRT can matter. For example, if you have your uterus, your ovaries, both or neither, if you have any pre-existing conditions, as well as your age. Even with age, it will depend on the type of estrogen, dose and why, and how, you are using it. For example vaginal estrogen is administered in such small doses that it is thought to carry almost no risks for most women. These are just some examples of why no one-size-fits-all.

What Type of HRT?

When it comes to HRT, there are various forms available, and it is crucial to find the right combination and dosage that works for you and you can choose how you want to administer your HRT —whether through a spray, patch, gel or pill. Generally speaking, it is always better to use body-identical hormones if you can.

The 2 main hormones used in HRT are:

- estrogen – types used include estradiol, estrone and estriol
- progesterone/progestin – either a synthetic version of the hormone progesterone - progestin - such as dydrogesterone, medroxyprogesterone, norethisterone and levonorgestrel, or a version called micronised progesterone (sometimes called body identical, or natural) that is chemically identical to the human hormone. Try to avoid medroxyprogesterone and choose micronised progesterone if you can.

HRT involves either taking both of these hormones (combined HRT) or just taking estrogen (estrogen-only HRT).

Estrogen-only HRT is usually only recommended if you have had your womb removed during a hysterectomy.

Regardless of the form, all types of HRT typically include estrogen, and if you have a uterus, and because estrogen can thicken the lining of the uterus (known as the endometrium), you need to take progesterone to prevent this. You may also need to replace your testosterone as well. It is essential to consider the type of HRT carefully and your dosage will depend upon the severity of your symptoms. Some women may require higher doses to achieve optimal results compared to others.

Progesterone can be in the form of body-identical progesterone, such as Utrogestan, Prometrium, Cyclogest, or Lutigest. Alternatively, a Mirena coil, which is a device inserted into the uterus to release hormones, can be used and it contains progestin.

Apart from contraception, the Mirena coil it is often used to manage heavy menstrual bleeding and typically contains a progestin hormone called levonorgestrel, making it a progesterone-only form of HRT. If it is used for menopausal symptoms, additional estrogen supplementation is required.

Estrogen is available in various forms, including pills, transdermal patches, gels and sprays, as well as vaginal rings, tablets, and creams.

The choice of transdermal HRT, which involves applying hormones directly to the skin, offers advantages.

Oral HRT

As the name suggests, oral HRT comes in the form of a pill and this is one of the most common forms of HRT. They are usually taken once a day.

Both estrogen-only and combined HRT are available as

tablets. For some women this may be the simplest way of having treatment.

Although the overall risk is small, it's important to be aware that there are some risks of oral HRT, and some of these were covered by the WHI study and it can also include blood clots,. The risks, with oral HRT tablets, however small, are higher than with transdermal HRT. This is due to the hormones being digested by the body and the supporting organs, particularly the liver (see below). Oral combined HRT that is commonly prescribed in the UK by the NHS also contains a progestin rather than progesterone and this is also very typical in many countries including the US. Ask your physician about trans-dermal HRT which is body identical.

Transdermal HRT

Transdermal HRT is a type of hormone replacement therapy that you use on your skin. It can be as a gel, patch or a spray and is typically applied to the forearm or inner thigh, but always applied to the skin. This means that it gets into your body directly through your skin and enters your blood. The good thing about this is that it doesn't go through your liver first, which can lead to fewer side effects and doesn't increase the (still low) risk of a blood clot or stroke.

On top of that, all types of f transdermal estrogen contains the body identical estrogen, $17\text{-}\beta$ estradiol. The progesterone used in transdermal HRT, as well as testosterone, is also body-identical and derived from yam.

The estrogen patch, gel or spray should be used continuously, without breaks, so there is a constant release of the hormone straight into your bloodstream. You can increase or decrease the amount you use which can be great when you are dealing with your hormone fluctuations during the peri menopause and as you move into menopause.

The progesterone used in transdermal HRT (and testosterone) is also body identical (derived from yam).

If you can, opt for transdermal HRT and request it from your health care professional.

Vaginal estrogen

Estrogen is also available as a cream, pessary or ring that is placed inside your vagina and it is used to help relieve vaginal dryness, but will not help with other symptoms such as hot flushes. It is very effective and considered safe for most women i.e the doses are so small that it does not increase your risk of breast cancer, so you can use it without taking progesterone, even if you still have a womb 9but always double check with your doctor).

Progesterone replacement

The way you take progesterone will depend on the kind you're using and whether you're still having periods. As noted above, if you're still getting periods, you'll usually take 200mg of Utrogestan or Prometrium each night for two weeks out of every month. Both are bioidentical hormones and research shows they have fewer side effects.

Once your periods have stopped, you'll usually take 100mg of Utrogestan or Prometrium each night. If you have side effects from progesterone, like feeling low, you can often use the capsules vaginally, or try a different kind of progesterone. These dosages are provided as an example and your healthcare provider will be know what is best for you.

The amount of progesterone you need doesn't always depend on how much estrogen you're taking. There isn't strong evidence to say that women on a higher dose of estrogen need a higher dose of progesterone. Some women are on a higher dose because their skin doesn't absorb estrogen as easily. Others need higher doses to help with their symptoms.

If you're having bleeding when you shouldn't be, you should talk to your healthcare provider. This might happen in the first 3-6 months after starting or changing your dose of HRT, and it can happen with both high and low doses of estrogen. Sometimes, taking a higher dose of progesterone can help with the bleeding.

In a recent study at Newson Health, less than 1% of their patients had abnormal vaginal bleeding and they couldn't find a link between the dose of estradiol and the chance of having this kind of effect.

At the time of writing, there is a shortage of supply of Utrogestan in the UK and, according to the manufacturers, this is due to exceptionally high demand. Although it is the only brand on the market in the UK which contains micronised progesterone alone there is a combination tablet – Bijuve – which combines micronised (bio-identical) progesterone with a body identical estrogen. However, because this contains oral estrogen it may not be suitable for everyone and you may be at higher risk of certain complications including Deep Vein Thrombosis (DVT) than the estrogen that can be absorbed through the skin.

Testosterone

Testosterone is available as a gel that you rub onto your skin. It is not currently licensed for use in women in the UK, but it can be prescribed after the menopause by a specialist doctor if they think it might help restore your sex drive.

Testosterone is usually only recommended for women whose low sex drive (libido) does not improve after using HRT and it is used alongside another type of HRT.

At the start of testosterone replacement, the dose is usually 5mg of cream or gel daily. After 3-6 months a blood test is done to check the level of testosterone and often also your sex hormone binding globulin (SHBG) to determine your Free Androgen Index (FAI).

If your levels are low despite treatment with testosterone and you are still experiencing symptoms of testosterone deficiency (reduced libido, low energy, reduced motivation) then you may be recommended to increase the amount of testosterone gel or cream you are using and then repeat the blood test again after a few months.

The side effects due to testosterone are very rare if levels of testosterone and Free Androgen Index remain in the female range but can include acne and unwanted hair growth.

HRT treatment routines

There are 2 types of routines are cyclical (or sequential) HRT and continuous combined HRT and these depend on whether you're in the early stages of the menopause or have had menopausal symptoms for some time.

Cyclical HRT

Cyclical HRT, also known as sequential HRT, is often recommended for women taking combined HRT who have menopausal symptoms but still have their periods.

There are 2 types of cyclical HRT

Monthly HRT

Monthly HRT is usually recommended for women having regular periods and with this type of HRT you take estrogen every day, and take progesterone alongside it for the last 14 days of your menstrual cycle.

3-monthly HRT

This is usually recommended for women having irregular periods, usually a period every 3 months. In this case you take estrogen every day, and take progesterone alongside it for around 14 days every 3 months.

This is a great example of when a diary can come in useful! It will help you log the frequency of your period more accurately - it is very easy to loose track of when you had your last one as you go through peri menopause.

Irregular bleeding is a common side effect in the first months of HRT use, particularly with continuous HRT and with three-monthly cyclical HRT. If it continues after the first three to six months its sensible to get this checked by your doctor.

Continuous combined HRT

Continuous combined HRT is usually recommended for women who are postmenopausal i.e. you have not had a period for 1 year and, as the name suggests it involves taking estrogen and progesterone, or estrogen-only HRT every day without a break.

We have so far explored a lot about hormone replacement therapy (HRT), including how it works, the different forms of hormones used, and the influence of factors such as your health status and timing of HRT initiation. It's crucial to recognize that all these elements contribute to shaping the best HRT plan tailored for you.

You should not have any periods while on continuous HRT if you were prescribed after you have been through the menopause.

Today, with advancements in research and medical science, women have a plethora of options for menopause treatment.

Alternatives to combined estrogen and progesterone HRT

1. Estrogen-only therapy (ET): This type of HRT involves the use of estrogen alone, without

progesterone. Estrogen-only therapy is generally recommended for women who have undergone a hysterectomy (surgical removal of the uterus) but is not used if you still have a womb (uterus).

2. Tibolone: Tibolone is a synthetic hormone that acts on estrogen, progesterone, and androgen receptors. It has estrogenic, progestogenic, and androgenic effects and is used to treat menopausal symptoms and prevent osteoporosis. Tibolone is sometimes used as an option for women who cannot use estrogen-based HRT.

3. Selective estrogen receptor modulators (SERMs): SERMs, such as raloxifene, are compounds that selectively bind to estrogen receptors and produce estrogen-like effects in some tissues while blocking estrogen activity in others. Raloxifene is primarily used to prevent and treat osteoporosis in postmenopausal women. If you have a have a uterus or womb then you need to take progesterone as well to protect against uterine cancer.

4. Low-dose vaginal estrogen: For women experiencing localized menopausal symptoms such as vaginal dryness and discomfort during intercourse, low-dose vaginal estrogen products, like creams, tablets, or rings, can be an effective alternative. These products deliver a small amount of estrogen directly to the vaginal tissues, which helps alleviate symptoms with minimal systemic absorption.

5. Non-hormonal options: For women who prefer to avoid hormonal treatments altogether, non-hormonal options like lifestyle changes, dietary adjustments, and over-the-counter or prescription medications can help manage menopausal symptoms. Examples include

regular exercise, consuming a balanced diet, and using lubricants for vaginal dryness.

Lifestyle, diet and natural remedies are covered in more detail in the following chapters but it's useful to include some alternative strategies here too.

To look at other forms of natural hormone therapy the Menopause Strategies: Finding Lasting Answers for Symptoms and Health (MsFLASH), tested multiple non-hormone treatments, completing five clinical trials involving more than 1,300 women in the U.S. They tested nine interventions to treat hot flashes, sleep problems, and other menopausal symptoms.

The results showed that cognitive behavioral therapy for insomnia improved sleep using six individual therapy sessions over an eight-week period, covering topics such as strengthening the association between bed and sleep and improving bedtime routines.

Non-hormonal medications were also studied. Two types of antidepressants — a selective serotonin reuptake inhibitor (SSRI) called escitalopram and a serotonin and norepinephrine reuptake inhibitor (SNRI) called venlafaxine — improved menopausal symptoms, including hot flashes and sleep problems. The SNRI showed similar effects to low-dose estradiol MHT for hot flashes.

Non-Hormonal Prescription Medications: Some non-hormonal medications can help alleviate certain menopausal symptoms. For instance, selective serotonin reuptake inhibitors (SSRIs), as mentioned in the above research, have been shown to reduce hot flashes. Other medications, such as Gabapentin and Clonidine, originally developed to treat conditions like epilepsy and high blood pressure respectively, have also shown some efficacy in relieving hot flashes.

Phytoestrogens

We have talked about phytoestrogens before and we will cover them again in the chapter on diet and natural remedies but basically phytoestrogens are plant-based compounds that behave like estrogen in the body.

Yam is the phytoestrogens that is used in transdermal HRT and Yam-based products, such as creams or supplements, are often marketed as "natural" alternatives to conventional hormone replacement therapy (HRT). These products are derived from wild yam and contain a compound called diosgenin, which can be chemically converted into progesterone or other hormones in a laboratory.

Firstly, it's essential to note that the human body cannot convert diosgenin from wild yam into hormones like progesterone or estrogen. This conversion requires a specific laboratory process, so simply consuming wild yam or applying a wild yam cream will not provide the same hormonal benefits as conventional HRT.

Some yam-based products claim to contain "natural progesterone" or "bioidentical hormones." While bioidentical hormones are chemically identical to the hormones produced by the human body, their safety and efficacy can vary depending on the specific formulation, dosage, and route of administration. All this means is that make sure you are dealing with a reputable brand and talk to your doctor.

According to the North American Menopause Society, The term "bioidentical hormone therapy" began as a marketing term for custom-compounded hormones. Since then it is used to mean hormones that have the same chemical and molecular structure as hormones produced by the body (body identical). Bioidentical hormones do not have to be custom-compounded (meaning custom mixed). But for this reason, double check whether bioidentical means body identical.

Interactive Exercise

1. Period tracker - keep a diary including when they start, end and include any symptoms even if you don't think they are related (feeling dizzy, migraines, energy levels etc)

2. Educate yourself - hopefully this book is just the start - to understand what is happening to your body.

3. Talk to people

Chapter Resources

Menopause Strategies: Finding Lasting Answers for Symptoms and Health (MsFLASH): https://www.fredhutch.org/en/research/divisions/public-health-sciences-division/research/cancer-prevention/msflash.html

NICE (2015) 'Menopause: diagnosis and management': www.nice.org.uk/guidance/ng23

British Menopause Society (2020): 'BMS & WHC's 2020 recommendations on hormone replacement therapy in menopausal women'

Tinhofer I.E., Zaussinger M., Geyer S.H., Meng S., Kamolz L.P., Tzou C.H., Weninger W.J. (2018), *'The dermal arteries in the cutaneous angiosome of the descending genicular artery'*, *J Anat*, 232(6) pp.979-86. doi: 10.1111/joa.12792.

Singh I., Morris A.P. (2011), *'Performance of transdermal therapeutic systems: effects of biological factors'*, *Int J Pharm Investig*, 1(1):4-9. doi: 10.4103/2230-973X.76721.

Liu, P., Higuchi, W.I., Ghanem, A.H., Good, W.R. (1994), *'Transport of beta-estradiol in freshly excised human skin in vitro: diffusion and metabolism in each skin layer'*, *Pharmaceutical Research*, 11(12), pp.1777–84. doi.org/10.1023/a:1018975602818

Leopold C.S, Maibach H.I, (1996), *Effect of lipophilic vehicles on in vivo skin penetration of methyl nicotinate in different races, International*

Journal   of   Pharmaceutics,   139,   1–2,   pp.161-67, doi.org/10.1016/0378-5173(96)04562-0.

NHS   Hormone   replacement   therapy   (HRT): https://www.nhs.uk/conditions/hormone-replacement-therapy-hrt/types/

Here are some well-known sources that explain the research behind the statement about micronised progesterone compared to synthetic progestin:

Progesterone and preterm birth: This study discusses the use of progestogens, including progesterone, for women at high risk of preterm birth. (https://pubmed.ncbi.nlm.nih.gov/32524598/)

Micronized vaginal progesterone to prevent miscarriage: a critical evaluation of randomized evidence: This review evaluates the effects of first-trimester use of vaginal micronized progesterone in preventing miscarriages.(https://pubmed.ncbi.nlm.nih.gov/32008730/)

The pharmacodynamics and safety of progesterone: This review discusses the unique pharmacodynamic activity and safety profile of natural progesterone compared to synthetic progestins. https://pubmed.ncbi.nlm.nih.gov/32739288/

Impact of micronised progesterone and medroxyprogesterone acetate in combination with transdermal oestradiol on cardiovascular markers in women diagnosed with premature ovarian insufficiency or an early menopause: a randomised pilot trial: This clinical trial compares the effects of micronised progesterone and medroxyprogesterone acetate on cardiovascular disease risk markers in women diagnosed with early menopause and premature ovarian insufficiency. https://pubmed.ncbi.nlm.nih.gov/35688490/

These sources provide evidence that micronised progesterone, which is identical to the hormone your body naturally produces, has been proven to be safer than its synthetic counterpart and has fewer side effects.

FOURTEEN

The Hormonal Diet to Tackle Weight Gain and Health

M enopause can bring about weight gain and changes in body shape, but with the right strategies and lifestyle adjustments, it is possible to maintain a healthy weight and feel fabulous during this phase of life.

There are a few reasons why you gain weight during menopause. For starters, muscles mass declines and this slows the rate that your body uses calories i.e. your metabolism slows. It means that if you are eating the same amount of calories, you won't burn them up as quickly. It's one of the reasons exercise helps - it both strengthens muscles and uses calories.

And did you know that the loss of estrogen can cause excess 'bad' fat in your abdomen and organs that can go on to cause obesity, Type II diabetes, and heart disease. HRT helps this.

There are other factors that can contribute to this that are triggered by menopause. Low mood can lead to comfort eating while some medications that might be prescribed at this time can also lead to weight gain. And then, of course, gaining weight can make you feel down and lower your self-esteem. It can be quite the negative cycle can't it?

And to add insult to injury, the falling estrogen, can increase inflammation in our joints and in our gut - and both can lead to weight gain.

Our dietary choices significantly influence the symphony of hormones within our bodies. Just as a string quartet without a cello or a choir missing its sopranos, certain foods can disrupt our hormonal balance. Conversely, a nutrient-dense and balanced diet can help fine-tune our body's hormonal rhythms.

Natural hormonal therapies are often used to address hormonal imbalances and include lifestyle changes such as diet and exercise, as well as the use of supplements and herbs (which we will discuss shortly).

During and after menopause, it becomes crucial to pay attention to your diet and lifestyle choices in order to support hormonal balance and overall health. Here are some key strategies to consider:

Limiting processed foods and added sugars: Excessive consumption of processed foods and added sugars can contribute to weight gain, inflammation, and hormonal imbalances. Instead, focus on whole, nutrient-dense foods to support your overall health.

Reducing alcohol consumption: Consuming alcohol excessively can interfere with hormone production and balance, and it also increases the risk of various health issues. It is advisable to consume alcohol in moderation or avoid it altogether.

Managing stress: Chronic stress can have a significant impact on hormonal balance and overall well-being. Incorporating stress management techniques such as meditation, yoga, or deep breathing exercises can help support hormonal balance and improve your overall health.

Staying active: Regular physical activity plays a crucial role in maintaining a healthy weight, supporting hormonal balance, and improving overall health. Aim to engage in a combination of cardiovascular and resistance training exercises most days of the week.

Let's begin by understanding the role of macronutrients, which include carbohydrates, proteins, and fats. Complex carbohydrates such as whole grains and legumes act as slow-burning fuel, providing sustained energy and helping regulate blood sugar levels. High-quality proteins from sources like lean meats, fish, eggs, or plant-based proteins like lentils and quinoa provide the building blocks for hormone production.

Healthy fats, especially omega-3 fatty acids found in fatty fish, walnuts, and flaxseeds, support cell health and help control inflammation.

In addition to macronutrients, micronutrients also play a crucial role in managing menopause symptoms. Calcium and vitamin D are essential for bone health, magnesium aids in sleep and mood regulation, and vitamin B6 supports liver function and hormone regulation.

It's also important to limit the intake of processed foods and sugars because they can disrupt the harmony and flow of your internal symphony, causing inflammation and contributing to conditions like insulin resistance and high cholesterol. Consider them as noise pollutants that interrupt the performance.

Hydration is another vital aspect of our diet that cannot be overstated. It aids in digestion, nutrient absorption, and detoxification processes. Aim for at least eight glasses of water a day, or more if you're active or live in a hot climate.

Next, let's address the role of the gut microbiome in hormone regulation. The gut can be likened to the backstage crew of our performance, working behind the scenes to keep the show running smoothly. A healthy gut aids in proper digestion and absorption of nutrients, as well as the detoxification of excess hormones. Probiotic foods such as yogurt, sauerkraut, and other fermented foods can support a healthy gut microbiome. Some strains of probiotics have been specifically linked to improved hormone health, such as Lactobacillus rhamnosus.

By now you will also be familiar with the key strategies, some of which is covered in the following chapter.

1. Reducing alcohol consumption: Excessive alcohol intake can interfere with hormone production and balance, as well as increase the risk of various health issues. It is advisable to consume alcohol in moderation or avoid it altogether.
2. Managing stress: Chronic stress can impact hormonal balance and overall health. Incorporating stress management techniques, such as meditation, yoga, or deep breathing exercises, can help support hormonal balance and well-being.
3. Staying active: Regular physical activity can help maintain a healthy weight, support hormonal balance, and improve overall health. Aim to engage in a combination of cardiovascular and resistance training exercises most days of the week.

Dietary strategies will go hand in hand with the lifestyle modifications we discussed earlier. Combining a balanced diet, regular physical activity, good sleep hygiene, and stress management techniques, you are conducting a symphony of wellness, where every note contributes to the harmony of menopause management.

The Importance of Nutrition for Hormonal Health

When you consider your diet, you are looking to lower blood sugar levels, boost your immune system and gut health to stimulate your microbiome, provide vitamins including C, D and

Magnesium and eat the 'good fats' to name just some of the essential needs.

Eating a diet rich in whole, nutrient-dense foods like fruits, vegetables, whole grains, and lean proteins can help regulate hormones, reduce inflammation, and support overall health and well-being.

Certain foods, like soy products, flaxseed, and legumes, contain phytoestrogens, compounds that can mimic the effects of estrogen in the body. If you still have your uterus then you need to include progesterone. If you have the cancer gene or have breast cancer then it's better to avoid estrogen unless it is for vaginal dryness (and applied topically in micro doses), just ensure you check with your doctor first.

Fats

Good Fat

Proper nutrition is crucial for hormonal health and this includes 'healthy' fats.

You might have heard that monounsaturated and polyunsaturated fats can work wonders for your hormone health, but do you know why? Let's break it down and explore how these types of fats impact certain hormones and why that matters for your overall well-being.

First up, let's clarify what monounsaturated and polyunsaturated fats are. These types of fats are considered "good fats" and they play a crucial role in maintaining a healthy, balanced diet.

Monounsaturated fats are found in foods such as olive oil, avocado, nuts, and seeds, and have been shown to help reduce inflammation, improve cholesterol levels, and support heart health.

Polyunsaturated fats, including omega-3 and omega-6 fatty acids, are found in foods such as fatty fish, nuts, seeds, and vegetable oils, and also have a range of health benefits. Omega-3 fatty acids, for example, have been shown to reduce inflammation, support brain health, and improve heart health, while omega-6 fatty acids are important for skin and hair health, and support immune function.

Now, let's talk hormones. Well, it turns out that monounsaturated and polyunsaturated fats can be pretty important for keeping them in check.

One hormone that loves these good fats is **insulin**. Produced by the pancreas, insulin is responsible for regulating your blood sugar levels. When you eat foods rich in monounsaturated and polyunsaturated fats, your body becomes more sensitive to insulin, which helps maintain stable blood sugar levels. This is particularly important for people with type 2 diabetes or those at risk of developing the condition. In fact, a 2018 study found that consuming more unsaturated fats was linked to a reduced risk of type 2 diabetes.

Next up is **leptin**, the famous "satiety hormone" that tells your brain when you've had enough to eat. Produced by your fat cells, leptin levels tend to be lower in people who are obese or overweight. Research suggests that eating a diet rich in monounsaturated and polyunsaturated fats can help regulate leptin levels, which can aid in weight management and appetite control.

Another hormone that benefits from these healthy fats is **cortisol**. Commonly known as the "stress hormone," cortisol is produced by the adrenal glands and plays a vital role in regulating our stress response. Too much cortisol, however, can lead to a whole host of issues, including weight gain, mood disorders, and inflammation. Monounsaturated and polyunsaturated fats have been shown to help reduce inflammation and lower cortisol levels, which can help support overall hormone health.

Now let's talk about **estrogen** and **progesterone**, the two primary female sex hormones. Believe it or not, monounsaturated and polyunsaturated fats can help support healthy estrogen and progesterone levels too! A study published in the Journal of Clinical Endocrinology and Metabolism found that women who consumed more monounsaturated fats had higher estrogen and progesterone levels, which can be particularly important during menopause when hormone levels naturally decline.

Not to be left out, we have **testosterone**, responsible for supporting muscle growth, bone density, and sex drive.

While testosterone is commonly known as the primary male sex hormone, it's also produced in smaller amounts in women's ovaries and adrenal glands. In fact, testosterone is essential for women's health, playing a vital role in maintaining bone density, muscle mass, and overall wellbeing.

Testosterone levels in women naturally decline as they age, particularly during menopause. This decline can lead to a range of symptoms, including loss of muscle mass, decreased libido, and reduced bone density, increasing the risk of osteoporosis. Some women may also experience symptoms of low testosterone, including fatigue, weight gain, and mood changes.

While testosterone replacement therapy is sometimes used to treat low testosterone in women, it's important to note that the optimal levels of testosterone for women are lower than those for men. This is because high levels of testosterone in women can lead to unwanted side effects, such as acne, facial hair growth, and a deeper voice.

There are several herbs and herbal remedies that may help support healthy testosterone levels in women. Here are a few examples:

1. **Maca root**: This adaptogenic herb has been used traditionally in South America to enhance fertility and libido. Some research suggests that maca may help increase testosterone levels in both men and

women, although more studies are needed to confirm this.

2. **Ashwagandha**: Another adaptogenic herb, ashwagandha has been shown to help reduce stress and anxiety, which can contribute to imbalanced hormone levels. Some research also suggests that ashwagandha may help increase testosterone levels in women with polycystic ovary syndrome (PCOS).

3. **Tribulus terrestris**: This herb has been traditionally used to enhance libido and fertility in both men and women. Some studies suggest that tribulus terrestris may help increase testosterone levels in women with low libido or sexual dysfunction.

4. **Fenugreek**: This herb is commonly used to enhance milk production in nursing mothers, but it may also have benefits for hormone balance. Some research suggests that fenugreek may help increase testosterone levels in women, although more studies are needed to confirm this.

5. **Rhodiola rosea**: This adaptogenic herb has been shown to help reduce stress and improve mood, which can support overall hormone balance. Some research also suggests that rhodiola may help increase testosterone levels in women.

As ever, it's important to note that while these herbs may have potential benefits for hormone balance and testosterone levels, more research is needed to fully understand their effects and potential side effects.

Overall, it's clear that including plenty of monounsaturated and polyunsaturated fats in your diet can have numerous health benefits, including supporting hormone regulation and overall wellbeing. So go ahead, enjoy that avocado toast or salmon dinner with confidence, knowing that you're doing something great for your body!

Bad Fat

Saturated and trans fats are considered to be unhealthy fats, particularly when it comes to hormonal health. These fats have been linked to increased inflammation, oxidative stress, and hormonal imbalances, all of which can contribute to a range of health problems.

Saturated Fat

Saturated and trans fats are considered unhealthy fats, especially when it comes to hormonal health. These fats have been linked to increased inflammation, oxidative stress, and hormonal imbalances, which can contribute to various health problems.

Saturated fats are commonly found in animal products such as meat, butter, and cheese, as well as in certain plant-based oils like coconut and palm oil. Consuming diets high in saturated fats has been associated with an elevated risk of heart disease, type 2 diabetes, and certain types of cancer. Some studies have also suggested that diets high in saturated fat may contribute to hormonal imbalances, particularly in women. For instance, research published in the Journal of Nutrition found that women who consumed diets high in saturated fat had lower levels of progesterone.

Coconut oil is a source of saturated fat, which has led to debates about whether it is a "good" or "bad" fat. While coconut oil is often promoted as a healthy alternative to other oils, research on its potential benefits and risks remains mixed.

Some studies have indicated certain health benefits of coconut oil. For example, research has found that the medium-chain triglycerides (MCTs) present in coconut oil may aid in weight loss, improve cognitive function, and reduce inflammation. Additionally, coconut oil has been suggested to possess antimicrobial properties that could potentially help fight infections (it can be useful for oil pulling and I sometimes use it for this purpose as well as for helping my dogs skin allergies in summer).

However, other studies have raised concerns about the potential negative effects of coconut oil on health. Some research has suggested that consuming coconut oil may elevate levels of LDL cholesterol, which can increase the risk of heart disease. A study published in the journal Nutrients found that diets high in coconut oil were associated with higher testosterone levels and lower progesterone levels in women, indicating a potential disruption in hormonal balance.

Therefore, while coconut oil may have some potential health benefits, it should not be relied upon as the sole source of dietary fat.

Trans Fats

Trans fats, also known as partially hydrogenated oils, are created when liquid oils are partially hydrogenated, or turned into solid fats.

These fats are are extremely unhealthy fats and have been linked to a range of health problems, including an increased risk of heart disease, type 2 diabetes, and certain types of cancer. Trans fats have also been shown to have negative effects on hormone balance and a study published in the Journal of the Academy of Nutrition and Dietetics found that diets high in trans fats were associated with lower levels of testosterone in men.

The American Heart Association recommends limiting saturated fat intake to less than 6% of daily calories, and avoiding trans fats altogether.

These fats are commonly found in many processed and fried

foods, as well as in baked goods and snack foods. Some examples of common foods that contain trans fats include:

Processed Foods:

- Margarine and other spreads
- Shortening and vegetable oils used in commercial baked goods
- Frozen dinners and meals
- Packaged snacks like crackers, chips, and popcorn
- Canned frosting and icing

Fried Foods:

- Fried chicken and other fried meats
- French fries and other fried potato products
- Fried doughnuts, pastries, and other baked goods
- Fried snack foods like onion rings and mozzarella sticks
- Fried fish and seafood dishes

Baked Goods:

- Commercially-prepared cakes, cookies, and other baked goods
- Pre-made pie crusts and pastries
- Frozen or pre-made dough for biscuits, cinnamon rolls, and other baked goods
- Some breads and crackers that are made with partially hydrogenated oils

Snack Foods:

- Packaged cookies and crackers

- Chips and pretzels
- Microwave popcorn
- Snack bars and granola bars

It's important to note that while some foods may be labeled as "trans fat-free," they may still contain small amounts of trans fats, so don't forget to read food labels carefully and choose whole, minimally processed foods whenever possible.

Protein

Protein is another essential nutrient for hormone production and balance. Protein sources like lean meats, poultry, fish, eggs, and legumes can help improve hormone balance. According to a review published in the Journal of the International Society of Sports Nutrition, protein plays a crucial role in hormone synthesis and secretion and can help improve hormone balance in both men and women.

Fibre

Fiber is also important for hormonal balance, as it can help regulate blood sugar and insulin levels. Foods that are high in fiber include fruits, vegetables, whole grains, and legumes. A study published in the Journal of Clinical Endocrinology and Metabolism found that higher fiber intake was associated with lower insulin levels in women with polycystic ovary syndrome (PCOS), a hormonal disorder that can cause menstrual irregularities and other symptoms.

Phytoestrogens are plant compounds that mimic the effects of estrogen in the body. Examples of phytoestrogen-rich foods include soybeans, flaxseeds, and lentils. A review published in the Journal of Steroid Biochemistry and Molecular Biology found that phytoestrogens can have a range of positive effects on hormonal health, including reducing menopausal symptoms and protecting against certain types of cancer.

Micronutrients like vitamins and minerals are also crucial for hormone production and balance. A review published in the journal Nutrients found that deficiencies in micronutrients like vitamin D, vitamin B12, and iron can negatively impact hormonal health and lead to a range of health issues. Foods that are rich in these micronutrients include leafy greens, nuts, seeds, and whole grains.

Sugar and Processed Foods

High sugar intake can disrupt hormonal balance and contribute to health issues like insulin resistance and metabolic syndrome.

Processed foods, which are often high in added sugars and unhealthy fats, can also disrupt hormonal balance and contribute to chronic disease.

A study published in the journal Nutrients found that high sugar intake was associated with increased insulin resistance and risk of PCOS in women. This suggests that reducing sugar intake can help support hormonal balance and prevent hormone-related health issues.

A diet high in processed foods has also been linked to hormonal imbalances and chronic disease. A study published in the journal Frontiers in Endocrinology found that a diet high in processed foods was associated with increased risk of metabolic syndrome and hormonal disorders like PCOS and thyroid disease.

The role of Insulin and Cortisol

High cortisol levels can also lead to weight gain, particularly around the abdomen, because it encourages the accumulation of fat cells in this area. It is why you might hear people talking about changes in fat distribution. This type of fat, known as visceral fat, is associated with a higher risk of metabolic and cardiovascular diseases.

High cortisol levels can also make it more difficult for our body to regulate blood sugar effectively. Cortisol increases glucose production in the liver and reduces insulin sensitivity in cells, making it more challenging for the body to maintain healthy blood sugar levels. This can increase the risk of developing type 2 diabetes, especially for women experiencing menopause-related hormonal imbalances.

Strategies for Balancing Blood Sugar and Insulin

Balancing blood sugar and insulin levels is crucial for hormonal health.

Eating a diet that is high in fiber, protein, and healthy fats can help improve insulin sensitivity and reduce the risk of insulin resistance and metabolic syndrome. For example, a study published in the journal Nutrients found that a diet high in fiber, protein, and healthy fats was associated with lower insulin levels and improved insulin sensitivity in women with PCOS.

Limiting sugar intake is also important for balancing blood sugar and insulin levels. Choosing whole, unprocessed foods like fruits, vegetables, whole grains, and lean proteins can help regulate blood sugar and reduce the risk of insulin resistance and metabolic syndrome.

Regular exercise is another effective strategy for balancing blood sugar and insulin levels. Exercise can help improve insulin sensitivity and reduce the risk of insulin resistance and metabolic syndrome. A study published in the journal Medicine and Science in Sports and Exercise found that regular exercise was associated with improved insulin sensitivity and lower risk of metabolic syndrome in women with PCOS.

Meal Planning for Hormonal Health

Building Hormone-balancing Meals

Meal planning can help ensure that you are consuming a variety of hormone-balancing foods and nutrients throughout the week. Building meals around a balance of macronutrients, including healthy fats, protein, and fiber, can help regulate blood sugar and support hormonal balance.

For example, a hormone-balancing breakfast might include a spinach and mushroom omelet with avocado and whole grain toast. This meal is high in protein, healthy fats, and fiber, which can help balance blood sugar and support hormone production and regulation.

A hormone-balancing lunch might include a grilled chicken salad with mixed greens, tomatoes, cucumbers, and a homemade dressing made with olive oil and apple cider vinegar. This meal is high in protein, healthy fats, and fiber, which can help regulate blood sugar and support hormonal balance.

A hormone-balancing dinner might include baked salmon with roasted sweet potatoes and Brussels sprouts. This meal is high in healthy fats, protein, and fiber, which can help regulate blood sugar and support hormone production and regulation.

Hormone-balancing Snacks and Treats

Healthy snacks can help keep blood sugar levels stable and provide important nutrients to support hormonal health. Some good options for hormone-balancing snacks include:

- Nuts and seeds: These are rich in healthy fats and protein, which can help regulate blood sugar and provide important nutrients for hormone production.

- Cut-up vegetables: Vegetables like carrots, celery, and cucumber are low in calories and high in fiber, which can help regulate blood sugar and provide important nutrients like vitamins and minerals.
- Fresh fruit: Fruit is a great source of fiber and antioxidants, which can support hormonal health and overall wellbeing.
- Yogurt or kefir: These dairy products are rich in protein and beneficial probiotics, which can help support gut health and hormonal balance.

Nourishing Foods to Your Plate for a Health Boost

Dietary improvements don't need to have strict and joyless rules that involve eliminating certain foods. Instead, consider incorporating these seven items into your meals, as recommended by chef, clinical nutritionist, and balance+ guru Emma Ellice-Flint. These simple, delicious, and affordable foods offer a wonderful nutritional boost during the perimenopause and menopause.

Turmeric: A Vibrant Spice with Multiple Benefits

Turmeric deserves a permanent place on our menus. It is rich in polyphenols, plant compounds that nourish and support the essential microbiota in our gut, offering a prebiotic effect. Maintaining the balance of these beneficial microorganisms becomes particularly important during the perimenopause and beyond since estrogen and testosterone, which also have anti-inflammatory effects, decline with age. This means it even more vital to seek out other sources of anti-inflammatory benefits.

Enjoy a nourishing drink by stirring a teaspoon of turmeric into warm milk or hot water. You can also mix it into a marinade for fish, a vinaigrette, or soup.

Seeds: Nutrient Powerhouses for Health

Seeds are an excellent alternative to nuts, offering a wide array of nutrients at a more affordable price. Despite their small size, these miniature heroes pack a punch of flavor and texture. They are rich in protein and omega-3 fatty acids, promoting heart health and reducing inflammation in the body. By reducing inflammation, you can potentially lower the risk of various inflammatory diseases, including cardiovascular disease, osteoporosis, Alzheimer's disease, clinical depression, and certain types of cancer. Seeds are also a great source of calcium and magnesium, essential for bone health and supporting mood and anxiety —important factors during menopause.

Add a generous amount of seeds onto your breakfast cereal, vegetable dishes, and soups.

Tinned Fish: A Convenient and Beneficial Addition

Oily fish is widely known for its nutritional value, but fresh fish can be expensive and environmentally unsustainable. Tinned fish is an excellent alternative to ensure you have a readily available source of goodness in your pantry. Affordable and with a long shelf life, it offers an impressive array of health benefits. Opt for varieties that include edible bones, such as sardines, pilchards, mackerel, anchovies, and certain brands of salmon. The bones of these fish provide a nutritional boost, with zinc and calcium promoting bone strength, while omega-3 fatty acids offer anti-inflammatory properties and protect against heart disease.

Ginger: Aid Your Digestion with a Natural Remedy

Whether in the form of fresh root or dried powder, ginger aids digestion by facilitating food movement in the gut. It acts as a prebiotic, nourishing the healthy microbiota in the gut, similar to the other foods on this list. Research suggests that the well-being and diversity of the microbiota in our gut significantly impact our overall health. By eating prebiotics found in ginger and other plant-based foods, we can enhance the anti-inflammatory effects of our gut microbes. During menopause, there is a decline in digestive enzymes and changes in gut microbes, which can potentially lead to digestive discomfort.

As well as using to flavor your food, ginger makes a great tea. Steep a couple of slices of fresh root or dried powder in boiling water.

Seaweed: A Nutrient-Rich, Underrated Option

Despite being surrounded by the sea, seaweed or sea vegetables are still not widely consumed in the UK or the US. They offer valuable prebiotic properties and are a good source of fiber, benefiting the gut microbiota. Seaweed is also rich in iodine, an essential mineral for thyroid gland function, supporting metabolism and energy production.

Rehydrate dried sea vegetables by soaking them in hot water for 10 minutes. Easily incorporate them into vegetable dishes, soups, or even add to natural yogurt.

Legumes: Affordable and Healthy Powerhouses

Lentils provide ample support for the gut microbiota and the gut lining that sustains these microbes, resulting in numerous anti-inflammatory benefits. Legumes are also excellent sources of protein, fiber, and minerals like calcium, magnesium, and iron.

Explore the variety of legumes available, including soy and chickpeas. Incorporating phytoestrogen-rich legumes can have a gentle effect on the body, helping alleviate some of the effects of declining estrogen during menopause (the effects are much milder than hormone replacement therapy).

The Role of Probiotics in Hormone Balance

Probiotics, known as "good" bacteria, play a vital role in digestive and overall health, and they also influence hormone balance. Research indicates that the gut microbiome, which comprises bacteria and microorganisms in our gut, can impact hormone levels and overall hormonal balance. By promoting the growth of beneficial bacteria and suppressing harmful bacteria, probiotics support a healthy gut microbiome.

Consider taking a probiotic supplement containing Lactobacillus acidophilus and Bifidobacterium bifidum.

Include fermented foods like yogurt, kefir, kimchi, kombuchand and sauerkraut in your diet - they are packed with probiotics - along with fiber-rich fruits, vegetables, and whole grains to support a healthy gut microbiome.

FIFTEEN

The Hormonal Lifestyle

In previous chapters, we have established that hormones are vital for our overall health and well-being, central to almost every function of our body. However, it's equally important to recognise the significant influence our lifestyle choices play in on our hormonal balance. This chapter will delve into the specific lifestyle factors that affect hormones and provide practical strategies for cultivating a lifestyle that complements hormonal health, along with examples for each effect or strategy.

Stress and Hormonal Health

Stress is an inevitable part of life, but chronic stress can wreak havoc on your hormonal health. When you experience stress, your body releases the hormone cortisol, the primary stress hormone, which can cause a host of problems if levels remain high for too long including weight gain, decreased immune function, and disturbed sleep

Along with high cortisol, chronic stress is linked to hormonal imbalances, including disrupted thyroid function and reduced levels of sex hormones like estrogen and testosterone.

The thyroid gland produces hormones that regulate the body's metabolism and energy levels. Chronic stress can interfere with thyroid function, leading to imbalances in thyroid hormone levels and potentially causing symptoms such as fatigue, weight gain, and mood changes.

Estrogen and progesterone, the primary female sex hormones, can also be affected. Chronic stress can lead to decreased levels of these hormones, potentially leading to menstrual irregularities, fertility issues, and other health concerns.

In addition to cortisol, thyroid hormones, and sex hormones, chronic stress can also impact insulin, the hormone responsible for regulating blood sugar levels. High levels of stress can lead to insulin resistance, which can contribute to the development of type 2 diabetes.

A study published in the Journal of Women's Health high-lighted that women reporting high stress levels also had higher cortisol levels and lower estrogen and progesterone levels. However, those who participated in stress-reduction activities such as yoga and meditation experienced lower cortisol levels and increased estrogen and progesterone levels, signifying the effectiveness of lifestyle interventions in restoring hormonal balance.

Another study published in the journal Metabolism found that chronic stress was associated with decreased thyroid function in women.

There are plenty of strategies you can use to manage stress and support your hormonal health.

Exercise and Hormonal Health

Regular exercise is crucial for hormonal balance. It helps regulate hormones like insulin and cortisol, essential for managing blood sugar and stress, respectively. Exercise also helps maintain healthy levels of sex hormones like estrogen and testosterone, particularly important for women approaching menopause.

The right levels of exercise (as well as a healthy diet) can protect against Type II Diabetes, cardiovascular disease and cancer and it can be particularly important during the peri menopause and menopause and here's why.

As we know from chapter 17, we lose around 10% of or bone mass during the first 5 years of menopause as bone breakdown outpaces bone growth. But exercise helps in a number of other ways:

1. Helps muscle strength which reduces during menopause
2. Exercises like yoga can help you de-stress and improve muscle strength
3. You are at more risk of cardiovascular disease during and after the menopause and regular exercise can protect agains this by improving cholesterol levels and managing blood pressure
4. Exercise can really help your mood because during exercise we release the feel-good chemicals, endorphines.
5. Falling estrogen can lead to changes in fat distribution around you body that often collects across around and below your waist.

However, not all exercise is created equal when it comes to hormonal health. High-intensity workouts and excessive exercise can actually lead to hormonal imbalances and other health issues.

For example, a study in the Journal of Endocrinology found that intense exercise can increase cortisol levels, causing weight gain, mood disorders, and inflammation. It can also decrease sex hormone levels in women, leading to irregular periods, decreased libido, and even infertility.

However, moderate exercises like walking, yoga, pilates, and low-impact cardio can have positive effects on hormone health.

For instance, strength training like weightlifting, yoga, and pilates can help improve muscle mass. Muscle tissues produce hormones like testosterone, and studies indicate that women who regularly engage in strength training have higher testosterone levels. Strength training can help increase levels of growth hormone, which is important for maintaining muscle mass and bone density. As well as this, it can help improve insulin sensitivity and reduce levels of cortisol. A study published in the journal Medicine and Science in Sports and Exercise found that strength training was associated with improvements in insulin sensitivity and glucose metabolism in postmenopausal women.

Walking is a simple, low-impact exercise that can be very beneficial for our hormonal health. A study published in the Journal of Endocrinology and Metabolism found that moderate-intensity walking can improve insulin sensitivity and lower levels of the stress hormone cortisol in overweight and obese women.

Aerobic exercises such as running, swimming, and cycling can positively impact mood, reducing symptoms of anxiety and depression, and regulate insulin levels, reducing the risk of developing insulin resistance, type 2 diabetes, and other metabolic problems.

Yoga is a great exercise for the whole body, not just muscle strength, that combines physical exercises (postures), breathing and meditation. It is widely reported by menopausal women to help with sleep, low mood, fatigue, and anxiety with some saying that it also helps reduce hot flashes as well as relieving aches and pains amd an help with symptoms of PMS and cramps. For many, it helps with clarity and focus. In fact, a 2013 study published in the Journal of Alternative and Complementary

Medicine found that a regular yoga practice can lead to significant improvements in menstrual pain and emotional well-being.

Alternate Nostril Breathing (Nadi Shodhana) is a breathing exercise associated with the beginning and end of yoga. It is used to help you relax and de-stress and can be helpful if you are having trouble sleeping.

To do this exercise simply :

1. Sit-up straight on a chair (or on the floor with your legs crossed). Take a few long breaths breathing through your nostrils then place your left arm on your left knee.
2. Use the thumb of your right hand to gently close your right nostril then inhale through your left nostril.
3. Once you have taken a breath, use the fourth ring finger (still using your right hand) to close your left nostril.
4. Release your thumb from your right nostril and exhale. Then inhale through your right nostril before closing it again.
5. Release your finger from your left nostril and exhale.

Repeat for a few minutes each day in the morning and the evening.

There are guidelines that say adults between the age 19 and 64 should be doing 30 minutes of moderate intensity exercise 5 times a week, with strength exercises on at least 2 days a week.

Techniques like deep breathing, meditation, and yoga can all help activate the parasympathetic nervous system, which is responsible for the body's rest-and-digest response. This can help decrease cortisol levels making you feel calmer and more relaxed.

Women have also had success with aromatherapy (the most popular choice is often Lavender or Rosemary and acupuncture.

Finally, let's not forget sleep and nutrition. Getting enough high-quality sleep is essential. Poor or insufficient sleep can affect hormones related to stress, appetite, and growth, among others. Try establishing a consistent sleep schedule, creating a relaxing sleep environment, and limiting screen time before bed, but also don't forget light.

You have special cells in your eyes that detect light and send signals to your brain which regulate the production of melatonin, the sleep hormone, and cortisol, our wakefulness hormone. An early morning walk can help regulate these hormones and improve sleep quality.

Try spending at least 15 to 30 minutes outside in the morning and again when the sun is high around 1-3pm. According to Dr xxxxx, during these times, your body naturally releases a little more melatonin, which can help with sleep later on.

If going outside is not possible, you can sit near a window or use lamps to add more light indoors, especially near your face. You are aiming to mimic natural light as much as you can because this can also help regulate your sleep-wake cycle.

You may also consider incorporating sleep-promoting supplements like magnesium or melatonin to support better sleep.

We have already covered aspects of diet and know that certain nutrients and dietary patterns can influence hormone production and function. For example, omega-3 fatty acids, found in fatty fish and some types of seeds, are known to reduce inflammation and help regulate hormones.

Daily Light Exposure, Vitamin D, and Hormonal Health

As well as helping with helping to maintain a balanced sleep-wake cycle, daylight helps in a number of other ways which the early morning walk can help with too.

Exposure to light also promotes the production of vitamin D, otherwise known as the "sunshine vitamin", which enhances the absorption of calcium and phosphorus from our food which are essential nutrients for muscle, teeth, and bone health.

Daylight can also help improve cognitive functions, alertness, mood regulation, and ward off anxiety and depression by increasing the release of the hormone serotonin.

Research also suggests that vitamin D can support the immune responses in our body, helping is to fight infections.

Sunlight exposure is also related to mood regulation and weight management and it triggers the release of serotonin, a hormone that boosts mood and brings about a sense of calmness. Studies show that exposure to daylight improves alertness, decision-making, cognitive function, and mood, helping to manage anxiety and depression.

When serotonin levels drop, the risk of depression increases, with some people experiencing a seasonal pattern to this mood lowering. In such cases, light therapy, or phototherapy, where light from a box mimics natural sunlight, can help stimulate serotonin production and decrease melatonin, the sleep-inducing hormone.

People with less daylight exposure may also notice changes in appetite, with cravings for high-carbohydrate foods leading to potential weight gain and energy depletion. It's thought that sunlight exposure levels can impact hunger hormones leptin and ghrelin, and daily time in sunlight may promote a healthier metabolism, body weight, and reduce the risk of type 2 diabetes.

Therefore, whenever possible, getting outside and facing the sun is a crucial aspect of self-care, whether for a walk or simply to enjoy your morning coffee.

The Importance of a Healthy Gut for Hormone Balance

The gut is where we absorb all the nutrients necessary for hormone production, and it also plays a vital role in eliminating excess hormones from the body. A healthy gut also ensures the proper production of serotonin, a hormone that regulates our mood and sleep patterns.

Research shows that certain types of bacteria in the gut microbiome, the community of beneficial bacteria living in our intestines, can affect the production of hormones like insulin, ghrelin (the hunger hormone), and leptin (the satiety hormone), among others.

Eating a diet rich in fibre, probiotics, and prebiotics can help support a healthy gut and support hormone balance. It's also important to avoid things that can harm the gut microbiome, such as chronic stress, lack of sleep, antibiotics (unless necessary), and a diet high in processed foods and sugar.

Of course, certain nutrients and dietary patterns can influence hormone production and function. For example, omega-3 fatty acids, found in fatty fish and some types of seeds, are known to reduce inflammation and help regulate hormones. We have covered much of this in the previous chapter.

Sleep Strategies

As with nutrition, we have dedicated a chapter to sleep (Tackling Tiredness) and it is worth reviewing that section. Getting enough high-quality sleep is also essential for your health and well-being and it is so often under-rated. Poor or insufficient sleep can affect hormones related to stress, appetite, and growth, among others.

Lifestyle Changes

Implementing certain lifestyle changes can significantly impact the severity and frequency of menopause symptoms. Regular exercise, maintaining a healthy weight, consuming a balanced diet, and avoiding triggers like caffeine and spicy foods can reduce hot flashes and improve sleep. It's also important to limit alcohol and quit smoking.

Mind-Body Techniques

Techniques such as yoga, tai chi, meditation, and deep-breathing exercises can help manage symptoms like mood swings, sleep disturbances, and hot flashes by reducing stress and promoting relaxation.

Over-the-Counter (OTC) Treatments:

Some nonprescription treatments can help manage specific symptoms of menopause. For example, vaginal lubricants and moisturizers can alleviate vaginal dryness, and cooling pads can help with night sweats.

Chapter Resources

Aranow C. (2021), 'Vitamin D and the immune system', J Investig Med, 59(6): pp.881-6. doi: 10.2310/JIM.0b013e31821b8755. PMID: 21527855; PMCID: PMC3166406.

Leppämäki S., Partonen T., Vakkuri O., Lönnqvist J., Partinen M., Laudon M. (2003), 'Effect of controlled-release melatonin on sleep quality, mood, and quality of life in subjects with seasonal or weather-associated changes in mood and behaviour', Eur Neuropsychopharmacol. 13(3): pp.137-45. doi: 10.1016/s0924-977x(02)00175-7.

Kripke DF. (2017), 'Light treatment for nonseasonal depression: speed, efficacy, and combined treatment', J Affect Disord. 217: pp. 90-96. doi: 10.1016/j.jad.2017.04.008.

Ríos-Hoyo A., Gutiérrez-Salmeán G. (2016), 'New dietary supplements for obesity: what we currently know', Curr Obes Rep. 5(2): pp.262-70. doi: 10.1007/s13679-016-0214-y.

Besedovsky L, Lange T, Haack M. The Sleep-Immune Crosstalk in Health and Disease. Physiol Rev. 2019;99(3):1325-1380. doi:10.1152/physrev.00010.2018).

SIXTEEN

Natural Remedies

There is a great deal of work going into natural and herbal remedies today, with many well-know women investing in this area - including Carrie Longton, the co-founder of Mumsnet.

A word of note here. Women who are living with estrogen positive receptive breast cancer and other types of cancer and illnesses are often excluded from many of the menopause aids including many of the phytoestrogen supplements. The current research on whether women with this condition need to avoid estrogen-mimicking effects like phytoestrogens is conflicting and, thankfully, much more is finally now being done.

I have written extensively on herbal and natural remedies including some of the reasons why we have so little historic research on their benefits, hopefully that is now being resolved - but it takes time. Not all herbs are good for you - but many more can really help.

They won't 'replace' your hormones but they can provide, if not similar support for your body, then they can at least relieve symptoms.

Top of this list is Soy. The Menopause Journal found that half a cup of soybeans a day reduced hot flashes by 79% (but the control group also saw a reduction of 49%). Mentioned elsewhere already, it contains phytoestrogen that helps release equol amd mimics the effect of estrogen in our body. It tends to work best for Asian women who have a slightly different gut microbiome which means they can digest it much more easily.

You can pick up Soy edamame beans in any large supermarket. Edamame beans are simply young green soybeans that are easy to cook and are the beans that that we eat more of as part of a meal.

Mature soybeans are harder and darker (yellow or brown) and tend to be used in cooking oil, tofu, miso, soy sauce and so on. They can also be soaked and used in soups, sauces and stews or dry roasted as a snack.

They both contain omega-3, are a complete source of protein and are packed with minerals - take note, mature soybeans contain more minerals than their younger edamame counterpart. They contain Iron, Potassium, Magnesium, Zinc, Copper, Manganese, Phosphorus and Selenium.

They area also both a rich source of Vitamin B containing Riboflavin, Vitamin B5, Vitamin B6 and Folate. Once again mature soybeans contain more of the these vitamins the immature edamame bean. In addition, soybeans and edamame contain small amounts of vitamins A, E and K.

Its an absolutely wonderful food and you should incorporate it into your diet in any case.

Also discussed elsewhere is Red Clover and it, too, has some evidence behind it in terms of helping manage hot flashes. Like Soy, it contains phytoestrogens, a plant compound that mimics the effects of estrogen. Its incredibly easy to incorporate into your daily routine - just pop a tea bag in a cup.

Nigella sativa, also known as kalonji or fennel flower, has flowers that produce antioxidant-rich seeds that contain thymoquinone. Studies have investigated the nigella seed's protective and therapeutic effects in those with polycystic ovarian syndrome (PCOS).

This seed may even provide an alternative to hormone replacement therapy (HRT) during menopause. This is still undergoing research, but it works by managing lower estrogen - the extract has been found to display estrogenic activity, meaning that it too, can act like estrogen in our body.

Other studies in animals have found that nigella seed extracts have helped regulate insulin, testosterone, luteinizing hormone, and thyroid hormone levels.

Concentrated Nigella sativa supplements are becoming increasingly popular and are also known as "black seed" or "black cumin seed." They are easy to add to bread, salads, and other dishes but, at the time of writing, the research is inconclusive and may have little of the benefits you hope for.

There is emerging work in the field of Nootropics, which is used to help focus, mental clarity and improve memory and is sometimes mentioned in relation to these menopause symptoms. Although there are numerous small studies that show nootropic supplements can positively affect the brain, there is, as of today, still not enough evidence from larger, controlled studies to know the effectiveness and safety of these in relation to peri menopause and menopause symptoms.

To a lesser degree, this is also true of CBD when it comes to menopause. Cannabidiol (CBD) is an active ingredient in cannabis that is derived from the hemp plant, but it doesn't cause a high and is not addictive. Research in the area around anxiety looks promising and CBD oil may well help those in peri menopause and who are waking up at night with a night sweat and a mind that can't calm down. The research isn't conclusive yet, but it is certainly one to try. It is better to start with 50mg capsules and work your way down to 10mg. Make sure you are buying from a reputable brand and check that the CBD has a batch number.

When it comes to maintaining hormonal balance, supplements and remedies can be a useful addition to a healthy diet and lifestyle. In the rest of this chapter, we'll highlight some of the most common hormone-balancing supplements and herbs, as well as vitamins, minerals, probiotics, teas, tonics, essential oils, aromatherapy, self-massage, and acupressure techniques that can support hormone health.

Supplements and Herbs

Supplements and herbs can be powerful allies in achieving hormonal balance. If you are buying as a store bought supplement then make sure that you check the amounts. Many contain so little of the herb that you need that it might not be worth the effort at all. Here are some common supplements and herbs that are known to support hormone health:

- Maca root: This Peruvian root is a popular adaptogen that is known to support the endocrine system. Maca root powder can be added to smoothies or used to make a hormone-balancing tonic. It is known to support healthy estrogen and progesterone levels, and can also help improve energy and mood.
- Ashwagandha: This adaptogenic herb is used in Ayurvedic medicine to support the adrenal glands and reduce cortisol levels, which can help to balance hormones and reduce stress helping and help sleeps. It can also support healthy thyroid function. It help with hot flashes, mood, memory. The best type of supplement is Organic Ashwagandha KSM-66. Ashwagandha tea or tincture can be consumed regularly to support overall hormonal health but don't

overuse, and always check dosage and conflicts with
other medications.

- Chaste tree berry: Also known as vitex, this herb is
  commonly used to support menstrual regularity and
  alleviate PMS symptoms. The berries were
  traditionally used during the menstrual cycle (and the
  early stages of menopause) to 'promote a healthy
  mind and body. It works by promoting healthy
  progesterone levels and reducing levels of prolactin, a
  hormone that can disrupt hormonal balance. Chaste
  berry tea or tincture can be consumed regularly to
  support hormonal health.
- Dong quai: A traditional Chinese herb that has been
  used for centuries to support female reproductive
  health and regulate the menstrual cycle.
- Black cohosh: This herb is commonly used to alleviate
  symptoms such as PMS, hot flashes and mood swings
  and can be good for the endocrine system. Be careful
  with black cohosh if you have any liver problems or
  have had cancer and definitely don't use this herb
  without consulting with a health professional.
- Red clover: This herb contains phytoestrogens, plant
  compounds that mimic the effects of estrogen in the
  body. Red clover tea can be a helpful addition to a
  hormone-balancing regimen, especially for women
  experiencing menopausal symptoms.
- Raspberry leaf: This herb is commonly used to
  support menstrual health and regulate menstrual
  cycles. It can also be helpful for women experiencing
  menopausal symptoms. Raspberry leaf tea can be
  consumed regularly to support hormonal health.
- Other extracts for the reproductive system include
  Damiana and Saw Palmetto, of of course St John's
  Wort.

In addition to herbs and supplements, vitamins and minerals also play a key role in hormonal health. Here are some of the most important ones to consider:

Vitamins and Minerals

Vitamin D is essential for overall health and is particularly important for hormonal balance. In fact, low levels of vitamin D have been linked to a variety of hormonal imbalances, including infertility and irregular menstrual cycles. While sunlight is the best source of vitamin D, it can also be found in fatty fish, egg yolks, and fortified foods.

Calcium is great for bone health and also plays a role in hormone regulation. Low levels of calcium have been linked to PMS and menstrual cramps. Good sources of calcium include dairy products, leafy greens, and fortified foods.

Adequate intake of vitamin D and calcium is important during childhood and adolescence when bones are growing and developing, and also during adulthood to maintain bone mass and prevent osteoporosis. Without enough vitamin D and calcium, bones may not form properly in childhood, and in adulthood, they can become weak and brittle, leading to an increased risk of fractures. It's worth noting that even if you consume enough calcium in your diet, your body won't absorb that calcium without enough vitamin D.

The mineral Magnesium is involved in over 300 different enzymatic reactions in the body and plays a crucial role in our hormonal health. It has been shown to improve insulin sensitivity, reduce inflammation, and lower cortisol levels. Good sources of magnesium include leafy green vegetables, nuts and seeds, and whole grains.

Zinc is another important mineral, and helps with the production of testosterone along with some other hormones. Low levels of zinc have been linked to menstrual irregularities and low libido in women. Good sources of zinc include oysters, beef, and pumpkin seeds.

The B vitamins, including B6, B12, and folate, are important for hormonal balance and overall health. They are involved in the production of neurotransmitters and hormones, and deficiencies in these vitamins have been linked to depression, anxiety, and menstrual irregularities. Good sources of B vitamins include leafy greens, whole grains, and animal products like meat and eggs.

Iron is essential for healthy blood flow and oxygen delivery, and is particularly important for women who lose iron during their menstrual cycle. Low levels of iron can lead to fatigue, mood swings, and decreased immune function. Good sources of iron include red meat, poultry, and leafy greens.

Selenium, a trace mineral is important for thyroid function and has been shown to improve mood and reduce inflammation. Good sources of selenium include Brazil nuts, seafood, and organ meats.

While vitamins and minerals can be helpful, it's always best to get them from whole foods rather than supplements whenever possible. This is because whole foods provide a variety of nutrients that work together, which can be more effective than taking isolated supplements.

Probiotics

We have talked about probiotics - the "good" bacteria that lives in our gut - in a recent chapter but it's worth repeating here because it is a good natural remedy. One study published in the journal Menopause by European Journal of Clinical Microbiology & Infectious Diseases found that taking a probiotic supplement containing Lactobacillus acidophilus and Bifidobacterium bifidum improved both vaginal and urinary symptoms in menopausal women.

In addition, and once again, as well as taking a probiotic

supplement, you can also support a healthy gut microbiome by eating fermented foods like yogurt, kefir, and sauerkraut, and by including plenty of fiber-rich fruits, vegetables, and whole grains in your diet.

Essential Oils

Essential oils are highly concentrated plant extracts that can be used for a range of health purposes, including supporting hormonal balance. These oils can be used in a variety of ways, including aromatherapy, topical application, and in some cases, ingestion.

One essential oil that is commonly used for hormonal health is clary sage. This oil is known to have estrogen-like properties and can help balance hormones in women experiencing menstrual irregularities, perimenopause, or menopause. It can be applied topically to the abdomen or diffused into the air for aromatherapy.

Another essential oil that is often recommended for hormone balance is lavender. This oil has been shown to help regulate cortisol levels, which can help reduce stress and support adrenal health. It can also be helpful for promoting relaxation and sleep, which can be beneficial for overall hormone balance.

Other essential oils that may be helpful for hormonal health include peppermint, fennel, geranium, and chamomile. Peppermint, for example, can help balance testosterone levels and support digestive health, while Geranium is known for its hormone-balancing properties that can be helpful for managing general menopausal symptoms.

It's important to note that essential oils should always be used with caution and under the guidance as they can be very potent and, like other herbs and supplements, may interact with medications or other health conditions.

Accupuncture, Self-massage and acupressure

Finally, let's talk about self-massage and acupressure techniques for hormonal balance. These practices involve using gentle pressure on specific points of the body to help promote circulation and balance energy and to manage stress, and alleviate symptoms like menstrual cramps and hot flashes . Some common acupressure points for hormone health include the inner ankle, the lower abdomen, and the point between the eyebrows.

- Spleen 6: This point is located on the inside of the leg, about three finger widths above the ankle bone. It is thought to help regulate menstrual cycles and alleviate PMS symptoms.
- Conception Vessel 6: Also known as the Sea of Energy, this point is located on the midline of the abdomen, about two finger widths below the belly button. It is thought to help regulate hormone levels and improve fertility.
- Kidney 3: This point is located on the inside of the ankle, just behind the ankle bone. It is thought to help regulate the menstrual cycle and improve energy levels.

To use these techniques, you can either use your fingers to apply gentle pressure to these points or use a tool like a massage ball or acupressure mat. It's important to note that while these practices can be helpful for promoting relaxation and reducing stress, they should not be used as a substitute for medical treatment.

Overall, there are many natural remedies and strategies that can be helpful for supporting hormonal health. Whether you choose to incorporate supplements, herbs, or lifestyle practices like yoga and meditation.

SEVENTEEN

Conclusion

W hen I finished writing this book I read it over a few times
and there was so much I wanted to add or change. So
much so, that I nearly held it back to re-write. I know I wanted to
say more about lots of things but mostly for women in their late
fifties, sixties and even seventies. I want to see more research on
this. There are some wonderful women in their late sixties who
swear by transdermal HRT. I wanted to say more about bone
health and heart disease, PCO ad PCOS and a number of
things. Each topic could be a book in its own right - and there are
indeed book out there dedicated to each area! PCO or PCOS?

In summary Poly Cystic Ovaries (PCO) is an indication that
there are more ovarian follicles than usual and can be seen in an
ultrasound scan where you would find over 12 ovaries and a
slightly enlarged ovary. PCO is very common and occurs in 20-
25% of all women of childbearing age. This is usually diagnosed
with an ultrasound scan (and best done by ultrasound scanning
through the vagina).

Meanwhile Poly Cystic Ovarian Syndrome (PCOS) is associated with the ovaries producing too many male sex hormones.

The diagnosis in this case means that you should have at least 2 (or 3) of the following:

- One or both ovaries must be polycystic.
- Long menstrual cycles of more than 35 days - or no menstruation.
- Signs of male sex hormone overproduction - this might display as increased hair growth and a blood test will clarify if this is the case.

I also wanted something factual, rather than 'woe is me' and I didn't want something that was too long! Yet, there is so much to say and so much research available. And I didn't want it to be too much of a depression session because we can help ourselves when we finally accept that it is simply biology. There is nothing 'bad' or 'wrong' with us, and life has so much to offer. Please, please read more on this subject and above all, talk. This should never be a subject to shy away from - because 90% of us women will all be affected in one way or anther.

When perimenopause strikes, most women are dealing with a myriad of life problems. Teenagers or empty-nest syndrome, aging parents, a heavy workload and on and on and on. For me it was, and is, aging parents and career. In the very early stages of perimenopause I was doing a start-up, I was what you would call a 'high flyer', at the peak of my career having been a director of a large company, then involved in a major sport club and, at that point, foraging my own path – or so I thought.

I now realise my reactions to lots of things were a result of my hormones changing my internal balance - erratically! I made some seriously bad choices at that time. I think the worst part was that I lost my confidence, and I let others take the lead or take over, even my own choices.

I don't regret that time - I hated it, but today, I don't regret where it lead.

As a result of those choices, I do what I do now. I live on an Island in a place that I love. I write books - I try to be the Orca ! Yes, life is not what I imagined it would be in my 20's and 30's. But here's the thing. It's better, it's more 'me'. I am happier within myself. I sometimes still hang on to the things I thought were important to my younger self, but I don't really think they were. They only mattered to what I thought others thought of me – they probably didn't and it wasn't the me I wanted, nor that I was.

And I have learned so much. I do seminars, coaching, conferences, masterminds – I love learning. And sometimes I get angry. I get very annoyed about healthcare – from dentistry (why do they put a known poison called mercury in our mouths), to the drugs we are provided that can only cause other problems, and why on earth do we still have 'one-size-fits-all' medicine when we know that mens' and womens' bodies work differently (as do the bodies of white people, black people and brown people).

The menopause effects half of the worlds population. We know what causes the problems both during and later in life – we know what can help. Yet still the available information is inadequate and not accessible. I was horrified to discover that some estrogen and progesterone products still carried out-dated medical leaflets in their packets that even the governing bodies of our health care providers know need up-dated. They are simply wrong - yet they still haven't 'got around' to doing it. After 5 years of more! Why is it that in the US and the UK (but not in France) healthcare providers still choose to dispense oral HRT with progestin and not transdermal HRT and progesterone. We know that is so much better! And we know, from that infamous WHI study that progestin is questionable.

HRT is not bad for you. Don't use estrogen-only if you have a uterus – you need progesterone too. Be careful with oral estrogen, especially if you have, or are susceptible to, breast cancer (but if you do and have vaginal dryness then the doses in the transdermal and pessaries are so small you should be ok – and they work). Choose body-identical and avoid progestin. Use herbs to support your health and your hormones. Don't trust the labels on everything you see on a shelf. Exercise with weight bearing if you can, swim, walk and try yoga. Look after your diet and include omega-3, soybeans (mature or immature!), and the other legumes. Don't forget your vitamins! And whatever you do look after you mental health, drink water and work on getting a good nights sleep. And that's it. It really is as simple as that.

Menopause is not the start of the last phase of your life. It offers the beginning of the one you dreamed of. It will be so much easier to get there if you recognise that there is help, you are not unusual and that most, if not all, of your symptoms and pain, really can be fixed. And they can. It's not rocket science. It's only basic biology. Just let your body top up on what it is needs.

But please, please read and research as much as you can too.

Here't to our magnificent 80's and 90's! What are you going to do?

Leave a review

Thank you for reading this book and I sincerely hope that you found it valuable. I would be eternally grateful if you would take just a few seconds to leave a review. You can leave a star rating or add some words.

Bibliography

Volek JS, Kraemer WJ, Bush JA, Incledon T, Boetes M. Testosterone and cortisol in relationship to dietary nutrients and resistance exercise. Journal of Applied Physiology. 1997;82(1):49-54.

Antonio J, Peacock CA, Ellerbroek A, Fromhoff B, Silver T. The effects of consuming a high protein diet (4.4 g/kg/d) on body composition in resistance-trained individuals. Journal of the International Society of Sports Nutrition. 2014;11(1):19.

Phelan N, O'Connor A, Kyaw Tun T, et al. Hormonal and metabolic effects of polyunsaturated fatty acids in young women with polycystic ovary syndrome: results from a randomized controlled trial. The American Journal of Clinical Nutrition. 2011;93(3):652-62.

Mense SM, Hei TK, Ganju RK, Bhat HK. Phytoestrogens and breast cancer prevention: possible mechanisms of action. Environmental Health Perspectives. 2008;116(4):426-33.

Oulhaj A, Jernerén F, Refsum H, Smith AD, de Jager CA. Omega-3 fatty acid status enhances the prevention of cognitive decline by B vitamins in mild cognitive impairment. The Journal of Alzheimer's Disease. 2016;50(2):547-57.

Fauser BC, Tarlatzis BC, Rebar RW, et al. Consensus on women's health aspects of polycystic ovary syndrome (PCOS): the Amsterdam ESHRE/ASRM-Sponsored 3rd PCOS Consensus Workshop Group. Fertility and Sterility. 2012;97(1):28-38.e25.

Alwosaibai A, Khoueiry R, Farah N, et al. Association between dietary patterns and metabolic syndrome in a sample of Lebanese adults. Frontiers in Endocrinology. 2019;10:384.

Asemi Z, Esmaillzadeh A. DASH diet, insulin resistance, and serum hs-CRP in polycystic ovary syndrome: a randomized controlled clinical trial. Hormone and Metabolic Research. 2015;47(3):232-8.

Vissers D, Hens W, Taeymans J, Baeyens JP, Poortmans JR, Van Gaal L. The effect of exercise on visceral adipose tissue in overweight adults: a systematic review and meta-analysis. PloS One. 2013;8(2):e56415.

Miller WL, Auchus RJ. The molecular biology, biochemistry, and physiology of human steroidogenesis and its disorders. Endocr Rev. 2011;32(1):81-151.

Storbeck KH, Swart AC, Swart P. Steroidogenesis: From cholesterol to DHEA. In: DHEA and the Intracellular Steroidogenesis. Elsevier; 2021. p. 1-17.

Davis SR, Lambrinoudaki I, Lumsden M, et al. Menopause. Nat Rev Dis Primers. 2015;1:15004.

Simons SS Jr, Chow CC. Steroid Hormones. In: eLS. John Wiley & Sons, Ltd; 2015.

Simpson ER, Clyne C, Rubin G, et al. Aromatase—a brief overview. Annu Rev Physiol. 2002;64:93-127.

Santoro N. The menopausal transition. Am J Med. 2005;118(Suppl 12B):8-13.

Stachenfeld NS. Hormonal changes during menopause and the impact on fluid regulation. Reprod Sci. 2014;21(5):555-561.

Prior JC. Progesterone for the prevention and treatment of osteoporosis in women. Climacteric. 2018;21(4):366-374.

Davis SR, Wahlin-Jacobsen S. Testosterone in women—the clinical significance. Lancet Diabetes Endocrinol. 2015;

Kicman AT. Pharmacology of anabolic steroids. Br J Pharmacol. 2008;154(3):502-521.

Nilsson O, Marino R, De Luca F, Phillip M, Baron J. Endocrine regulation of the growth plate. Horm Res. 2005;64(4):157-165.

Riggs BL, Khosla S, Melton LJ 3rd. A unitary model for involutional osteoporosis: estrogen deficiency causes both type I and type II osteoporosis in post-menopausal women and contributes to bone loss in aging men. J Bone Miner Res. 1998;13(5):763-773.

Rhen T, Cidlowski JA. Antiinflammatory action of glucocorticoids--new mechanisms for old drugs. N Engl J Med. 2005;353(16):1711-1723.

Whirledge S, Cidlowski JA. Glucocorticoids, stress, and fertility. Minerva Endocrinol. 2010;35(2):109-125.

Mullur R, Liu YY, Brent GA. Thyroid hormone regulation of metabolism. Physiol Rev. 2014;94(2):355-382.

Coutinho AE, Chapman KE. The anti-inflammatory and immunosuppressive effects of glucocorticoids, recent developments and mechanistic insights. Mol Cell Endocrinol. 2011;335(1):2-13.

Barnes PJ. How corticosteroids control inflammation: Quintiles Prize Lecture 2005. Br J Pharmacol. 2006;148(3):245-254.

Chrousos GP. Stress and disorders of the stress system. Nat Rev Endocrinol. 2009;5(7):374-381.

Smith SM, Vale WW. The role of the hypothalamic-pituitary-adrenal axis in neuroendocrine responses to stress. Dialogues Clin Neurosci. 2006;8(4):383-395.

Ulrich-Lai YM, Herman JP. Neural regulation of endocrine and autonomic stress responses. Nat Rev Neurosci. 2009;10(6):397-409.

Sapolsky RM. Stress, the Aging Brain, and the Mechanisms of Neuron Death. MIT Press; 1992.

McEwen BS. Protective and damaging effects of stress mediators: central role of the brain. Dialogues Clin Neurosci. 2006;8(4):367-381.

Patel TB, Du Z, Pierre S, Cartin L, Scholich K. Molecular biological approaches to unravel adenylyl cyclase signaling and function. Gene. 2001;269(1-2):13-25.

Avis NE, Crawford SL, Greendale G, et al. Duration of menopausal vasomotor symptoms over the menopause transition. JAMA Intern Med. 2015;175(4):531-539.

Freedman RR. Menopausal hot flashes: Mechanisms, endocrinology, treatment. J Steroid Biochem Mol Biol. 2014;142:115-120.

Maki PM, Kornstein SG, Joffe H, et al. Guidelines for the evaluation and treatment of perimenopausal depression: summary and recommendations. Menopause. 2018;25(10):1069-1085.

Manolagas SC, O'Brien CA, Almeida M. The role of estrogen and androgen receptors in bone health and disease. Nat Rev Endocrinol. 2013;9(12):699-712.

Mendelsohn ME, Karas RH. Molecular and cellular basis of cardiovascular gender differences. Science. 2005;308(5728):1583-1587.

Wenger NK. You've come a long way, baby: cardiovascular health and disease in women: problems and prospects. Circulation. 2004;109(5):558-560.

Maki PM, Henderson VW. Hormone therapy, dementia, and cognition: the Women's Health Initiative 10 years on. Climacteric. 2012;15(3):256-262.

Simpson ER. Sources of estrogen and their importance. J Steroid Biochem Mol Biol. 2003;86(3-5):225-230.

Stanczyk FZ, Clarke NJ. Advantages and challenges of mass spectrometry assays for steroid hormones. J Steroid Biochem Mol Biol. 2010;121(3-5):491-495.

Schindler AE. Progesterone and progestins: a general overview.

Silverberg SJ, Bilezikian JP. Evaluation and management of primary hyperparathyroidism. J Clin Endocrinol Metab. 1996;81(6):2036-2040.

Riggs BL. The mechanisms of estrogen regulation of bone resorption. J Clin Invest. 2000;106(10):1203-1204.

Carter CS, Pournajafi-Nazarloo H, Kramer KM, et al. Oxytocin: Behavioral associations and potential as a salivary biomarker. Ann N Y Acad Sci. 2007;1098:312-322.

Gouin JP, Carter CS, Pournajafi-Nazarloo H, et al. Marital behavior, oxytocin, vasopressin, and wound healing. Psychoneuroendocrinology. 2010;35(7):1082-1090.

Phillips SM. Dietary protein requirements and adaptive advantages in athletes. Br J Nutr. 2012;108 Suppl 2:S158-167.

Simopoulos AP. Omega-3 fatty acids in inflammation and autoimmune diseases. J Am Coll Nutr. 2002;21(6):495-505.

Pisoschi AM, Pop A. The role of antioxidants in the chemistry of oxidative stress: A review. Eur J Med Chem. 2015;97:55-74.

Aggarwal BB, Yuan W, Li S, et al. Curcumin-free turmeric exhibits anti-inflammatory and anticancer activities: Identification of novel components of turmeric. Mol Nutr Food Res. 2013;57(9):1529-1542.

Weaver CM, Alexander DD, Boushey CJ, et al. Calcium plus vitamin D supplementation and risk of fractures: An updated meta-analysis from the National Osteoporosis Foundation. Osteoporos Int. 2016;27(1):367-376.

Lustig RH, Schmidt LA, Brindis CD. Public health: The toxic truth about sugar. Nature. 2012;482(7383):27-29.

Shield KD, Parry C, Rehm J. Chronic diseases and conditions related to alcohol use. Alcohol Res. 2013;35(2):155-173.

Cornelis MC, El-Sohemy A, Campos H. Genetic polymorphism of the adenosine A2A receptor is associated with habitual caffeine consumption. Am J Clin Nutr. 2007;86(1):240-244.

Lovejoy JC. Weight gain in women at midlife: The influence of menopause. Obesity Management. 2009;5(2):52-56.

Ehrhart-Bornstein, M., & Bornstein, S. R. (2008). Hormones and the Endocrine System. In Encyclopedia of Neuroscience (pp. 1889–1901). Springer.

Gimpl, G., & Fahrenholz, F. (2001). The oxytocin receptor system: structure, function, and regulation. Physiological Reviews, 81(2), 629-683.

Smith, S. M., & Vale, W. W. (2006). The role of the hypothalamic-pituitary-adrenal axis in neuroendocrine responses to stress. Dialogues in Clinical Neuroscience, 8(4), 383.

Pearce, E. N. (2012). Thyroid hormone and obesity. Current Opinion in Endocrinology, Diabetes, and Obesity, 19(5), 408-413.

Gold, P. W. (2015). The organization of the stress system and its dysregulation in depressive illness. Molecular Psychiatry, 20(1), 32-47.

Mullur, R., Liu, Y. Y., & Brent, G. A. (2014). Thyroid hormone regulation of metabolism. Physiological Reviews, 94(2), 355-382.

Santin, A. P., & Furlanetto, T. W. (2011). Role of estrogen in thyroid function and growth regulation. Journal of Thyroid Research, 2011, 875125.

Kvetnansky, R., Sabban, E. L., & Palkovits, M. (2009). Catecholaminergic systems in stress: structural and molecular genetic approaches. Physiological Reviews, 89(2), 535-606.

Goldstein, D. S. (2010). Adrenal responses to stress. Cellular and Molecular Neurobiology, 30(8), 1433-1440.

Felger, J. C., & Treadway, M. T. (2017). Inflammation effects on motivation and motor activity

A 2019 review of clinical studies found that oral collagen supplementation could improve skin elasticity, hydration, and dermal collagen density. This suggests that collagen supplements might be beneficial for menopausal women experiencing a decline in skin health (source: https://pubmed.ncbi.nlm.nih.gov/30681787/).

A 2015 study on postmenopausal women showed that a daily oral intake of hydrolyzed collagen significantly increased skin elasticity compared to a placebo group (source: https://pubmed.ncbi.nlm.nih.gov/23949208/).

A 2018 study found that oral collagen supplementation in combination with other skin-nourishing ingredients (such as vitamins and antioxidants) led to significant improvements in skin elasticity, hydration, and wrinkle depth in postmenopausal women (source: https://pubmed.ncbi.nlm.nih.gov/29614461/).

Alberto Conegliani Barbosa, Maria do Carmo Gouveia Peluzio, Patrícia Borges de Oliveira, et al., "Effect of Lactobacillus acidophilus and Bifidobacterium bifidum supplementation to standard triple therapy on Helicobacter pylori eradication and dynamic changes in intestinal flora," European Journal of Clinical Microbiology & Infectious Diseases 34, no. 12 (2015): 2377-2386.

The Vaginal Microenvironment: The Physiologic Role of *Lactobacilli* Emmanuel Amabebe and Dilly O. C. Anumba* https://www.ncbi.nlm.nih.gov/pmc/articles/PMC6008313/

NICE (2015) 'Menopause: diagnosis and management', www.nice.org.uk/guidance/ng23

British Menopause Society (2020), 'BMS & WHC's 2020 recommendations on hormone replacement therapy in menopausal women'

Tinhofer I.E., Zaussinger M., Geyer S.H., Meng S., Kamolz L.P., Tzou C.H., Weninger W.J. (2018), 'The dermal arteries in the cutaneous angiosome of the descending genicular artery', *J Anat*, 232(6) pp.979-86. doi: 10.1111/joa.12792.

Singh I., Morris A.P. (2011), 'Performance of transdermal therapeutic systems: effects of biological factors', *Int J Pharm Investig*, 1(1):4-9. doi: 10.4103/2230-973X.76721.

Liu, P., Higuchi, W.I., Ghanem, A.H., Good, W.R. (1994), 'Transport of beta-estradiol in freshly excised human skin in vitro: diffusion and metabolism in each skin layer', *Pharmaceutical Research*, 11(12), pp.1777–84. doi.org/10.1023/a:1018975602818

Leopold C.S, Maibach H.I, (1996), Effect of lipophilic vehicles on in vivo skin penetration of methyl nicotinate in different races, *International Journal of Pharmaceutics*, 139, 1–2, pp.161-67, doi.org/10.1016/0378-5173(96)04562-0.

Menopause Strategies: Finding Lasting Answers for Symptoms and Health (MsFLASH): https://www.fredhutch.org/en/research/divisions/public-health-sciences-division/research/cancer-prevention/msflash.html

NHS Hormone replacement therapy (HRT): https://www.nhs.uk/conditions/hormone-replacement-therapy-hrt/types/

Treatment of menorrhagia during menstruation: randomised controlled trial of ethamsylate, mefenamic acid, and tranexamic acid: British Medical Journal, *BMJ* 1996;313:579 https://doi.org/10.1136/bmj.313.7057.579

Menopause Transition and Cardiovascular Disease Risk: Implications for Timing of Early Prevention: A Scientific Statement From the American Heart Association
https://www.ahajournals.org/doi/10.1161/CIR.0000000000000912

Aranow C. (2021), 'Vitamin D and the immune system', J Investig Med, 59(6): pp.881-6. doi: 10.2310/JIM.0b013e31821b8755. PMID: 21527855; PMCID: PMC3166406.

Leppämäki S., Partonen T., Vakkuri O., Lönnqvist J., Partinen M., Laudon M. (2003), 'Effect of controlled-release melatonin on sleep quality, mood, and quality of life in subjects with seasonal or weather-associated changes in mood and behaviour', Eur Neuropsychopharmacol. 13(3): pp.137-45. doi: 10.1016/s0924-977x(02)00175-7.

Kripke DF. (2017), 'Light treatment for nonseasonal depression: speed, efficacy, and combined treatment', J Affect Disord. 217: pp. 90-96. doi: 10.1016/j.jad.2017.04.008.

Ríos-Hoyo A., Gutiérrez-Salmeán G. (2016), 'New dietary supplements for obesity: what we currently know', Curr Obes Rep. 5(2): pp.262-70. doi: 10.1007/s13679-016-0214-y.

Besedovsky L, Lange T, Haack M. The Sleep-Immune Crosstalk in Health and Disease. Physiol Rev. 2019;99(3):1325-1380. doi:10.1152/physrev.00010.2018).

General Reading sources

NICE: National Institute of Healtcare and Excellence (https://www.nice.org.uk/)

A governmentally-run institute which provides "essential information for key groups including GPs, local government, public health professionals, social care professionals and members of the public".

British Menopause Society

https://thebms.org.uk

Royal College of Obstetricians and Gynaecologists

https://www.rcog.org.uk/for-the-public/menopause-and-later-life/

Newson Health or The Balance app

https://www.newsonhealth.co.uk

National Institute on Aging - What Is Menopause?

NIA leads a broad scientific effort to understand the nature of aging and to extend the healthy, active years of life. NIA is the primary federal agency supporting and conducting Alzheimer's disease research.

https://www.nia.nih.gov/health/what-menopause

Menopause Journal from the North American Menopause Society.

Menopause, published monthly, provides a forum for new research, applied basic science, and clinical guidelines on all aspects of menopause. You can read the summary of articles online https://www.menopausejournal.com and https://www.menopause.org/

https://www.health.harvard.edu/blog/menopause-and-memory-know-the-facts-202111032630

Made in the USA
Las Vegas, NV
28 October 2023